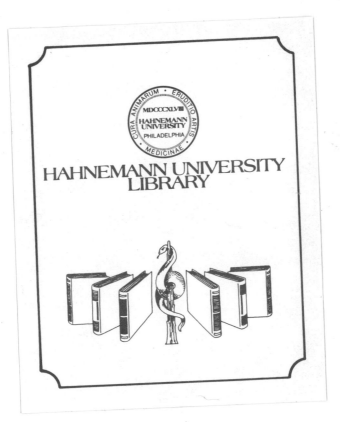

Raynaud's Phenomenon

Raynaud's Phenomenon

JAY D. COFFMAN
Boston University
School of Medicine

New York   Oxford
OXFORD UNIVERSITY PRESS
1989

Oxford University Press

Oxford   New York   Toronto
Delhi   Bombay   Calcutta   Madras   Karachi
Petaling Jaya   Singapore   Hong Kong   Tokyo
Nairobi   Dar es Salaam   Cape Town
Melbourne   Auckland

and associated companies in
Berlin   Ibadan

Library of Congress Cataloging-in-Publication Data

Coffman, Jay D. (Jay Denton), 1928–
Raynaud's phenomenon.

Includes bibliographies and index.
1. Raynaud's disease.   I. Title.
[DNLM: 1. Raynaud's Disease.   WG 570 C675r]
RC700.R38C63   1989   616.1′31   89–8578
ISBN 0-19-505756-2

1 2 3 4 5 6 7 8 9

Printed in the United States of America

To my wife, Louise,
and to the mentors
who most influenced my career:
Drs. Donald Gregg,
Robert W. Wilkins,
and J. Edwin Wood III.

Acknowledgments

The final completion of this book would not have been possible without the long hours of skillful work by Katherine Boris, who typed the entire manuscript. Marie Ryan was indispensable in gathering materials and making charts. I gratefully acknowledge Richard A. Cohen's constructive criticism and scientific insight. Grants from the National Heart, Lung, and Blood Institute for many years have funded the research and supported my interest in Raynaud's phenomenon.

Contents

Introduction

Raynaud's phenomenon is the occurrence of episodic attacks of well demarcated blanching or cyanosis of one or more digits on exposure to cold. Diffuse paleness or a bright red color of the digits and hands may occur on intense cold exposure in normal subjects. The distinguishing features of Raynaud's phenomenon are the episodic attacks, the white or blue color change confined to part or all of the digits, and the involvement of sometimes only a few digits. The prognosis is good for patients with the primary disease, with a few patients developing ulcerations or gangrene. However, when the phenomenon is due to an underlying disease, there may be multiple episodes of painful digital ulcerations or gangrene and systemic involvement affecting the length of life.

Primary Raynaud's disease and Raynaud's phenomenon secondary to one of several underlying etiologies are common medical problems. General practitioners and internists should be knowledgeable about the implications of vasospastic attacks of the digits, as the primary disease occurs in approximately one of six young women. Physicians must know which patients can be reassured and who to refer for special treatment. Secondary Raynaud's phenomenon touches almost all specialties including rheumatology (connective tissue diseases), hematology (cryoproteinemias, cold agglutinins), oncology (carcinomas), nephrology (dialysis patients), cardiology (emboli, β-adrenoceptor blockers), orthopedic surgery (thoracic outlet and carpal tunnel syndromes), occupational medicine (traumatic vasospastic disease), endocrinology (hypothyroidism), neurology (nerve entrapment syndromes), and dermatology (these physicians are often the first to see patients with connective tissue disease). Specialists must be aware of the diseases in their fields that cause Raynaud's phenomenon in order to institute a proper diagnostic work-up and treatment course.

Although Maurice Raynaud is credited with describing Raynaud's phenomenon in 1888, Davis (1982) suggested that the first description may have been in the Bible. In Exodus 12, Moses was commanded by the Lord to put his hand into his bosom, and when he withdrew it the hand was white as snow. He was told to put his hand back into his bosom, and when he withdrew it the hand was normal. Davis pointed out that Moses was in a cold area and was under great emotional strain. It is possible that these factors precipitated the vasospastic attack.

Raynaud's phenomenon and disease were not popular themes for investigation during the early twentieth century. In 1901 Hutchinson presented evidence that vasospastic attacks could have multiple etiologies and suggested the term *Raynaud's phenomenon* instead of *Raynaud's disease.* It was not until 1932 that Allen and Brown enumerated minimum criteria to differentiate primary Raynaud's disease from Raynaud's phenomenon due to secondary causes. The careful studies of Sir Thomas Lewis in 1929 indicated the presence of a local sensitivity to cold of the digital blood vessels. It was not until 1957 that Peacock supplied supporting evidence for the excess sympathetic activity theory expounded by Raynaud. A long lapse in interest then followed probably due to a lack of diagnostic tests and successful treatment modalities. During the last two decades there has been a resurgence of interest among investigators and pharmaceutical companies. This reawakening was predictable, as Raynaud's phenomenon is a common entity whose pathophysiology, diagnosis, and treatment are poorly understood. Pharmaceutical firms developed new classes of drugs for the treatment of coronary artery vasospasm and hypertension that relaxed small blood vessels. Because there was a large population of patients with Raynaud's phenomenon and adequate therapy did not exist, the firms also studied the use of these agents for this entity. New interest was stimulated in the pathophysiology and treatment of the syndrome by vascular specialists and rheumatologists owing to the introduction of calcium blocking agents, thromboxane synthetase inhibitors, angiotensin-converting enzyme inhibitors, serotonergic antagonists, and prostaglandins. Attempts to define diagnostic tests for the disease and the phenomenon have proliferated. Another reason for the renewed interest in vasospastic disease of the digits was the documentation that ischemic heart disease also could be caused by coronary vasospasm. The impetus to study the mechanism of vasospasm in the coronary arteries spread to the other, more accessible area involved by vasospastic attacks: the digits.

In this text, I have attempted to gather together much of what is known about primary Raynaud's disease and the secondary phenomenon. The primary aim was to collect in one place the present understanding of the physiology of finger blood flow and knowledge of the pathophysiology, etiologies, diagnosis, and treatment of primary and secondary Raynaud's phenomenon. Two closely related diseases, acrocyanosis and livedo reticularis, are also described, as they involve vasospasm and are important in the differential diagnosis of Raynaud's phenomenon.

The anatomy of the circulation of the hands and fingers is described in the first chapter. This subject is important to understanding how tissues survive when some of the blood vessels are obstructed. It may also help discern the location of the defect that produces a digit with well demarcated ischemia. The physiology of the finger circulation is then discussed. Mechanisms of vasoconstriction, including the sympathetic nerves and the α-adrenoceptors, local cold, and serotonin, may be pertinent to the pathophysiology of Raynaud's phenomenon. Mechanisms of vasodilation may also be important in vasospastic diseases, as defective vasodilation could enhance vasoconstrictor stimuli. For example, the β-blocking agents may induce Raynaud's phenomenon by inhibiting normal β-adrenoceptor vasodilation. Finally, there is a discussion of the techniques used to measure blood flow so that the reader may evaluate investigations described in this and later chapters.

The clinical picture and demographics of primary Raynaud's disease are described in Chapter 2. Prevalence studies, which are few in number, are presented. Prognosis, which is important to the physician when advising his patients, is also covered here. The pertinent points about prognosis are the excellent outlook for patients with the primary disease and the meaning of abnormal laboratory studies in a patient with Raynaud's phenomenon alone and no systemic manifestations of secondary disease.

Chapter 3 contains a short description of the pathology of primary Raynaud's disease. It is short because studies are scarce. There is little evidence that pathological abnormalities are present in the early stages of the primary disease. Angiographic studies of the blood vessels of the forearm, hand, and fingers are presented in this chapter because they can add to our knowledge of the pathology. However, there is no conclusive evidence that abnormalities exist in the primary disease.

Chapter 4 presents studies on the pathophysiology of primary Raynaud's disease. The evidence for the two classic theories of excessive sympathetic nervous system activity and a local fault in the digital arteries are considered. Investigative studies favor the latter theory and suggest that the defect may be at the α-adrenoceptor site. Other possible mechanisms involving the β-adrenoceptors, corticosteroids, histaminergic receptors, platelets, blood viscosity, cold vasodilatation, and serotonin are discussed. Evidence for the involvement of serotonin is strongest, at least for perpetuating if not actually inducing attacks. Finally, this material is summarized to illustrate how several of the factors discussed could act together to produce digital artery closure during cold exposure.

Chapter 5 notes that episodic attacks of well demarcated color changes of the digits on exposure to cold suffices for the diagnosis of Raynaud's phenomenon. Criteria are presented to rule out the secondary causes of Raynaud's phenomenon so as to arrive at the diagnosis of the primary disease. Objective tests are described that help in the diagnosis of Raynaud's phenomenon but not in the diagnosis of the primary disease. The most valuable are measurement of the digital systolic blood pressure following a general and local cold stimulus with digital ischemia and examination of the nailfold capillary bed.

The extensive number of secondary causes of Raynaud's phenomenon are discussed in Chapter 6. The commonest causes—drug therapy, connective tissue diseases, traumatic vasospastic disease, carpal tunnel syndrome, and thoracic outlet syndromes—are covered in detail, as it is possible that clues from their mechanisms may lead to a better understanding of the pathophysiology of the primary disease.

The various treatments that have been used for primary and secondary Raynaud's phenomenon are presented in Chapter 7. The calcium entry blocking agents and drugs that inhibit the sympathetic nervous system have been most extensively studied and are the most beneficial. Direct-acting vasodilators have not been successful in the treatment of vasospasm. Newer agents that inhibit thromboxane A_2, serotonin, or angiotensin and the vasodilator prostaglandins are discussed, although some of these agents are not yet available. Behavioral treatment/conditioning is explored and has been found to be an innocuous treatment that is helpful in some patients. A variety of other modalities are also discussed, most of which have little use in the treatment of Raynaud's phenomenon. The pros and cons of surgical sympathectomy conclude this chapter followed by a personal recommendation for treatment.

The final chapter describes two little understood diseases, acrocyanosis and livedo reticularis. Each may be associated with Raynaud's phenomenon, whether primary or secondary in etiology. It is important for the physician to be able to differentiate acrocyanosis from Raynaud's phenomenon because the prognosis and response to treatment may be different. Livedo reticularis, often present as a benign manifestation of primary Raynaud's disease, is frequently associated with the connective tissue diseases; however, it can also be a disabling form of vasculitis.

REFERENCES

Allen EV, Brown GE: Raynaud's disease: a critical review of minor requisites for diagnosis. *Am J Med Sci* 183:187, 1932.

Davis E: Raynaud's phenomenon of Moses. *Adv Microcirc* 10:110, 1982.

Hutchinson J: Raynaud's phenomenon. *Med Press Circ* 23:403, 1901.

Lewis T: Experiments relating to the peripheral mechanism involved in spasmodic arrest of the circulation in the fingers, a variety of Raynaud's disease. *Heart* 15:7, 1929.

Peacock JH: Vasodilatation in the human hand: observations on primary Raynaud's disease and acrocyanosis of the upper extremities. *Clin Sci* 17:575, 1957.

Raynaud M: *On Local Asphyxia and Symmetrical Gangrene of the Extremities.* Translated by T. Barlow. London: The Syndenham Society, 1888, p. 99.

Raynaud's Phenomenon

1

Anatomy and Physiology of Finger Circulation

Knowledge about the anatomy of the arterial circulation of the hand and digits is important to the understanding of some facets of Raynaud's phenomenon. The presence of two digital arteries and dorsal digital arteries often prevents ulcers or gangrene when only one digital vessel is obstructed. The thumb is often spared during vasospastic attacks, probably because its blood vessels arise directly from the radial artery and not the palmar arch.

The hand and fingers are supplied by the ulnar and radial arteries. In the palm there are two arches: (1) the superficial palmar arch, supplied by both the superficial branch of the radial artery (although it is variable) and the end branch of the ulnar artery; and (2) the deep palmar arch, formed by the deep branch of the ulnar artery and the end of the radial artery. Infrequently the median artery, a large branch of the anterior interosseous artery, joins the deep palmar arch. The superficial palmar arch lies under the midpalmar fascia, and the deep palmar arch is located dorsal to the flexor tendons on the palmar interosseous fascia. The two digital arteries to the third through fifth fingers and the ulnar side of the second finger are supplied by the superficial palmar arch via common digital arteries. The digital arteries of the thumb and radial side of the index finger usually derive from a branch of the radial artery (the princeps pollicis). The deep palmar arch gives off metacarpal arteries, which supply dorsal digital arteries, which in turn anastomose with the common digital arteries.

Whether the ulnar artery or the radial artery is the predominant blood supply to the palmar arches and the digits, and if the palmar arches form a complete bridge between the ulnar and radial arteries, assume importance in obstructions of the arteries at the level of the wrist. These occlusions occur in the hypothenar hammer syndrome and in connective tissue diseases. For instance, with an ulnar artery occlusion and an incomplete superficial palmar arch, severe digital ischemia usually occurs. The ulnar artery is larger at the elbow but smaller than the radial artery at the wrist in postmortem anatomical studies (Keen, 1961). However, when the two vessels are measured using a doppler ultrasonic probe, there is no difference in their diameter at the wrist (Doscher et al., 1983). If the superficial palmar arch continues to show normal flow by doppler examination during occlusion of the radial or ulnar artery, the arch is considered complete. Morphological and physiological studies differ markedly in gauging its completeness. In an anatomical study (Coleman and Anson, 1961), 21.5 percent of 650 hands had incomplete arches, whereas an angiographic study reported this figure to be 66.3 percent (Varro et al., 1978). However, in doppler flow studies, only 9 to 11 percent of arches appeared to be incomplete (Doscher et al., 1983; Little et al., 1973). In these studies it was determined that the ulnar artery blood flow was usually dominant.

ARTERIOVENOUS ANASTOMOSES

The circulation of the human digits is complex compared to those for other cutaneous vascular beds. In addition to the capillary circulation, the finger contains a large number of arteriovenous (A-V) anastomoses (Fig. 1–1), which are coiled blood vessels with thick muscular walls that are supplied with many nerve endings. They directly connect the arterial with the venous circulation, bypassing the capillary beds. Although investigators differ, A-V shunts are reportedly most numerous in the nail bed ($501/cm^2$ of surface area), tips of digits ($236/cm^2$), and palmar surface of the digits ($20-150/cm^2$) (Grant and Bland, 1931). Some are present in the palm of the hand and the sole of the foot, but they are almost absent from the dorsum of these areas. They have also been described in the human ear (Prichard

Fig. 1–1. Circulation of the fingertip showing the dual circulation of the capillary bed and the large number of arteriovenous anastomoses. The thick arrows indicate that most stimuli have a greater vasoconstrictor or vasodilator effect on the arteriovenous anastomoses than the capillary bed. *Source:* Coffman and Cohen (1988c).

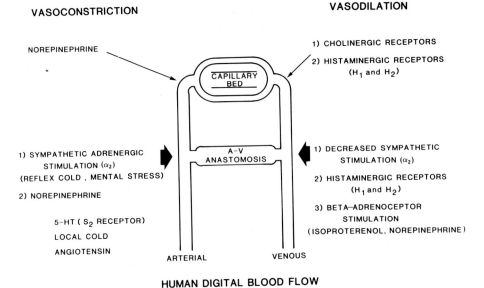

VASOCONSTRICTION　　　　　　　　　　　　　　VASODILATION

NOREPINEPHRINE

1) CHOLINERGIC RECEPTORS

2) HISTAMINERGIC RECEPTORS
(H$_1$ and H$_2$)

CAPILLARY BED

1) SYMPATHETIC ADRENERGIC
STIMULATION (α_2)
(REFLEX COLD , MENTAL STRESS)

2) NOREPINEPHRINE

5-HT (S$_2$ RECEPTOR)
LOCAL COLD
ANGIOTENSIN

A-V
ANASTOMOSIS

1) DECREASED SYMPATHETIC
STIMULATION (α_2)

2) HISTAMINERGIC RECEPTORS
(H$_1$ and H$_2$)

3) BETA–ADRENOCEPTOR
STIMULATION
(ISOPROTERENOL, NOREPINEPHRINE)

ARTERIAL　　　　　　　VENOUS

HUMAN DIGITAL BLOOD FLOW

and Daniel, 1956). These shunts are important in the regulation of body temperature, opening in warm environments to allow increased blood flow to dissipate body heat or closing during cold exposure to save body heat. For this reason, fingertip blood flow varies from less than 1 ml·min^{-1} 100 ml^{-1} of tissue to approximately 180 ml·min^{-1} 100 ml^{-1} of tissue (Greenfield and Shepherd, 1950). They are mainly under the control of the sympathetic nervous system (Coffman, 1972). A high concentration of cholinesterase has also been shown to be present by histochemical studies (Hurley and Mescon, 1956). It may be pertinent that Raynaud's phenomenon affects only skin areas that possess A-V shunts; hence perhaps this fact should continue to be an area of investigation to determine the pathophysiology of Raynaud's phenomenon.

CENTRAL CONTROL OF FINGER BLOOD FLOW

The integration and regulation of the circulation including finger blood flow is accomplished in the hypothalamus, medulla oblongata, and spinal cord. The hypothalamus regulates flow through the cutaneous A-V anastomoses to control body temperature and blood pressure; emotional responses also occur through this center. The hypothalamus receives messages from most other higher centers in the cerebral cortex to coordinate its function. The medulla oblongata contains the pressor and depressor vasomotor centers. They are strongly influenced by the hypothalamus but must also integrate messages from the baroreceptors, chemoreceptors, and somatic afferent nerves. The medullary centers communicate with the peripheral vessels by means of the sympathetic vasoconstrictor nerves. Messages from the medulla travel in the spinal cord in the intermediolateral cell columns to the sympathetic ganglia and then to the nerves. Lesions or malfunction at any of these central levels may lead to peripheral disturbances of vasomotor control of the digital blood vessels.

MECHANISMS OF DIGITAL VASOCONSTRICTION

Sympathetic Nervous System and Digital Blood Flow

Digital blood flow is decreased by activation of the sympathetic nerves and increased by withdrawal of their activity. This process is evidently the primary mechanism of vasoconstriction and vasodilation in the digits. Reflex sympathetic vasoconstriction by body cooling or application of cold to other parts of the body results in intense digital vasoconstriction, which is absent in sympathectomized limbs. Digital nerve block results in a large digital blood flow due to the absence of sympathetic activity. In this discussion, total finger blood flow was measured by venous occlusion plethysmography and capillary flow by the disappearance rate of a radioisotope from a local injection in the pad of the fingertip.

In vitro experiments using hand arteries and veins have shown that α_1- and α_2-adrenoceptors are present by using pharmacological antagonists and agonists.

The population of adrenoceptors is evidently heterogeneous in digital arteries and veins (Stevens and Moulds, 1981). For example, prazosin, an α_1-adrenoceptor antagonist, does not affect norepinephrine contraction in digital artery strips, whereas it inhibits the response in veins (Jauernig et al., 1978). There are many other dissimilarities between hand arteries and veins in reaction to adrenoceptor agonists and antagonists in in vitro studies. It has also been shown that proximal digital artery strips are more sensitive to α_1- than α_2-adrenoceptor antagonists, whereas distal digital arteries need both adrenoceptor antagonists to prevent their contraction in response to norepinephrine (Flavahan et al., 1987). Similarly, the distal digital arteries are more sensitive to α_2- than α_1-adrenoceptor agonists. In man, intraarterial phenylephrine (0.2–1.3 µg/min), an α_1-adrenoceptor agonist, and clonidine (0.12–0.48 µg/min), an α_2-adrenoceptor agonist, produced dose-related decreases in total finger blood flow and increases in vascular resistance (Coffman and Cohen, 1988a) (Fig. 1–2). Prazosin, an α_1-adrenoceptor antagonist, effectively blocked the vasoconstrictor effect of phenylephrine but not that of clonidine, and yohimbine, an α_2-adrenoceptor antagonist, blocked the effect of clonidine but not that of phenylephrine. During reflex sympathetic vasoconstriction produced by body cooling, yohimbine produced a significant increase in finger blood flow and a decrease in vascular resistance, whereas prazosin had no significant effect (Fig. 1–3). No changes occurred in finger capillary flow with yohimbine or prazosin. Thus α_1- and α_2-adrenoceptors are present in human digital vasculature, and α_2-adrenoceptors are more important than α_1-adrenoceptors during reflex sympathetic vasoconstriction. The α_2-adrenoceptors predominantly affect A-V shunts in the finger.

　　In normal subjects during reflex sympathetic vasoconstriction produced by body cooling, total finger blood flow significantly decreases, and capillary blood flow is not affected (Coffman, 1972) (Fig. 1–4). Therefore the A-V shunts must have

Fig. 1–2.　　Dose-related decreases in total fingertip blood flow (plethysmography) with intraarterial infusions of the α_1-adrenoceptor agonist phenylephrine and the α_2-adrenoceptor agonist clonidine. *Source:* Coffman and Cohen (1988a).

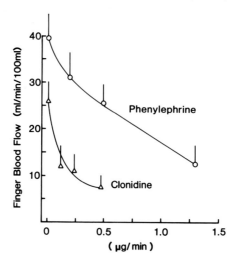

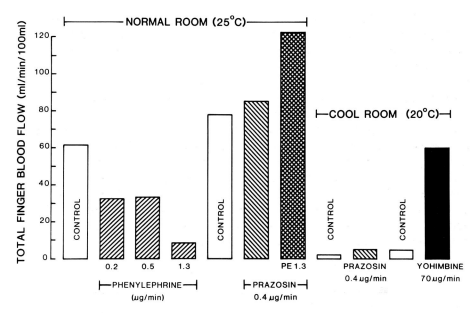

Fig. 1–3. Total fingertip blood flow measured by venous occlusion plethysmography in one normal subject. In the 25°C room, phenylephrine decreased blood flow, and prazosin inhibited the effect of the largest dose of phenylephrine, indicating that α_1-adrenoceptors were blocked. During reflex sympathetic vasoconstriction induced by body cooling, the same dose of prazosin produced only a small increase in blood flow, whereas yohimbine greatly increased flow, indicating that α_2-adrenoceptors are more important than α_1-adrenoceptors in sympathetic neural vasoconstriction. *Source:* Coffman and Cohen (1988a).

constricted while nutritional blood flow was maintained, which would be an appropriate way for the digits to help regulate body temperature. The sympathetic neurotransmitter norepinephrine, administered intraarterially, was also shown to significantly decrease total finger blood flow but caused a small decrease in capillary flow. An estimate of A-V shunt flow by subtraction of capillary from total flow indicates that 80 to 90 percent of finger flow is shunted during vasodilation. During vasoconstriction the shunt flow may be small. The A-V shunts can vary the blood flow of the digits over a wide range in order to dissipate or save body heat and evidently are primarily controlled by the sympathetic nervous system via α_2-adrenoceptors.

It has been shown that there is a regular rhythm of spontaneous periods of vasoconstriction in the fingers of 30 seconds to 2 minutes when subjects are in a comfortable environment. If the environment becomes warmer, the interval increases between periods of vasoconstriction. From these findings, Burton and Taylor (1940) surmised that there was a continuous reflex adjustment of peripheral blood flow to regulate body temperature that consists in a modification of vascular tone that has intrinsic rhythmicity. Using the laser–doppler technique, Engelhart and Kristensen (1986) observed rhythmic fluctuations of finger flow, with a frequency of five to ten per minute, and irregular fluctuations superimposed on the

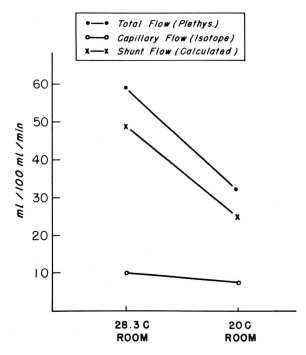

Fig. 1–4. Total fingertip blood flow (measured by venous occlusion plethysmography) and capillary blood flow (measured by the disappearance rate of a local depot of radioisotope) were measured in normal subjects before (28.3°C room) and during (20°C room) reflex sympathetic nerve stimulation (total body cooling). With body cooling, the decrease in capillary blood flow was not significant, but the total and arteriovenous shunt flow were decreased significantly.

rhythmic fluctuations. The irregular fluctuations increased with cooling. The rhythmic variations continued, but the irregular fluctuations disappeared in nerve-blocked fingers or sympathectomized limbs.

Finger blood flow decreases rapidly at the onset of bicycle exercise and is maintained at low levels for the duration of the exercise (Kitamura et al., 1982); however, the decrease in finger blood flow does not correlate with the intensity of the exercise. Superficial veins of the hand and forearm also constrict in response to exercise under normal thermal conditions (Rowell et al., 1971). Heating the skin markedly attenuates or abolishes the venomotor response, and cooling restores it. Because of the rapidity with which the venomotor changes occur and the lack of correlation with changes in right atrial temperature, investigators have suggested a reflex mechanism initiated via cutaneous thermoreceptors.

Heat Vasoconstriction

Nagasaka and co-workers (1986) observed vasoconstriction when fingers were heated in a waterbath to a temperature of 39° to 40°C. No comparable response was found in the forearm skin. They suggested that it may be a mechanism to reduce heat gain through the hand when skin temperature rises above core body temperature and that the A-V anastomoses are probably important in the response. The mechanism of this vasoconstriction was not investigated.

Serotonin

In vitro pharmacological studies have demonstrated the presence of S_2-serotonergic receptors in human hand arteries and veins (Arneklo-Nobin and Owman, 1985). They can be stimulated by 5-hydroxytryptamine (5-HT) and antagonized by ketanserin, an S_2-serotonergic blocking agent. Roddie and co-workers (1955) found that intraarterial 5-HT (4–16 μg/min) decreased forearm and hand blood flow in normal subjects; finger blood flow (calorimetric technique) decreased with 5-HT 16 μg/min in the one subject studied. 5-HT produced an increase in forearm and hand volume as well as a deep red color. In normal subjects in our laboratory (Coffman and Cohen, 1988b), intraarterial 5-HT (4 and 8 μg/min) decreased total finger blood flow in a dose-related manner, whereas 2 μg/min had no effect. 5-HT also decreased finger capillary blood flow. A reddening of the distal limb and hand occurred with active doses. The effect of 5-HT was blocked by ketanserin. Because ketanserin also has α_1-adrenoceptor antagonist activity, prazosin was given in doses that blocked phenylephrine, an α_1-adrenoceptor agonist, during reflex sympathetic vasoconstriction produced by body cooling in normal subjects. Prazosin had no effect on finger blood flow. Ketanserin (50 μg/min) then produced a large increase in finger blood flow and blocked the effect of vasoconstrictor doses of 5-HT (Fig. 1–5). These experiments indicate that 5-HT receptors are present in the digits and that their blockade by ketanserin during reflex sympathetic vasoconstriction leads to vasodilation. Angiotensin and clonidine, an α_2-adrenoceptor agonist, were shown still to have a vasoconstrictor effect during ketanserin infusions, proving that the vasodilation was not nonspecific (Fig. 1–6). Phentolamine increased finger blood flow during ketanserin, and ketanserin increased flow during yohimbine infusions, also indicating that α_2-adrenoceptors were not involved. This study indicates that S_2-serotonergic receptors may be another important mechanism of vasoconstriction in the digit. However, it has yet to be shown that serotonin is present during sympathetic vasoconstriction in the digits. The source could be the platelets, or there may be serotonergic nerves, as have been demonstrated in cerebral blood vessels (Griffith et al., 1982).

LOCAL COLD AND COLD VASODILATATION

Local cooling decreases fingertip blood flow but usually not to as great an extent as reflex sympathetic vasoconstriction. For example, environmental cooling at 20°C decreased blood flow to 8.9 ml·min^{-1} 100 ml^{-1} in eight normal subjects. Following

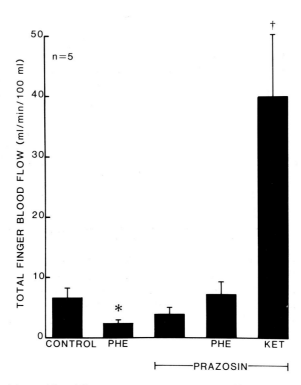

Fig. 1–5. Total finger blood flow (mean ± SEM) measured by venous occlusion plethysmography is shown for five normal subjects during reflex sympathetic vasoconstriction produced by body cooling. Intraarterial phenylephrine (PHE) significantly decreased finger blood flow (*$p < 0.05$) before but not during α_1-adrenoceptor blockade during prazosin infusion. Ketanserin (KET), during prazosin, produced a large, significant increase in finger blood flow (†$p < 0.025$). *Source:* Coffman and Cohen (1988b).

digital nerve blockade, blood flow rose to 74 ml; local cooling of the finger then decreased blood flow to 49 ml (Cohen and Coffman, unpublished observations) (Fig. 1–7). The mechanism of the vasoconstriction with local cooling is unknown but may involve increased sensitivity of receptors to the effect of circulating or locally released humoral agents.

If a finger is cooled at less than 10°C for 15 minutes, blood flow almost ceases, but then the temperature of the skin of the finger rises to about 28°C; nonimmersed adjacent fingers remain cooler (Greenfield and Shepherd, 1950; Lewis, 1930; Marshall et al., 1953). The temperature of the finger then fluctuates slowly with periods of vasoconstriction, alternating with vasodilatation; this process is called the *hunting reaction* (Fig. 1–8). The intensity of the cold vasodilatation parallels the number of A-V anastomoses in the skin (Grant and Bland, 1931). It occurs in the human fingers and toes, ear lobes, and nose tip but not in the skin of the forearm,

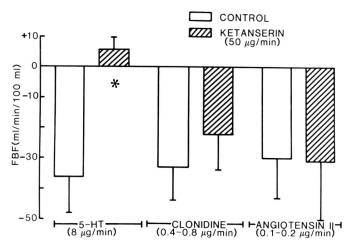

Fig. 1-6. Changes in total finger blood flow (mean ± SEM) induced by 5-hydroxy-tryptamine (5-HT), clonidine (an α_2-adrenoceptor agonist), and angiotensin II before (white bars) and during (hatched bars) ketanserin infusion. Only the change in finger blood flow caused by 5-HT was significantly different during ketanserin (*$p < 0.05$), demonstrating the specificity of the S_2-serotonergic blockade. *Source:* Coffman and Cohen (1988b).

Fig. 1-7. Total fingertip blood flow (plethysmography) measured during environmental cooling to induce reflex sympathetic vasoconstriction (left bar) in eight normal subjects. Following digital nerve anesthesia to block the sympathetic nerves, there is a large increase in blood flow (middle bar). Local cooling of the fingertip then caused a significant decrease in blood flow (right bar). The lines through the bars indicate standard deviations from the mean blood flow. *Source:* Cohen RA, Coffman JD: unpublished observations.

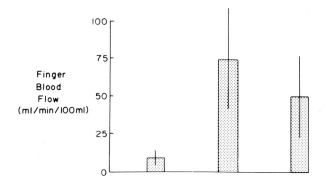

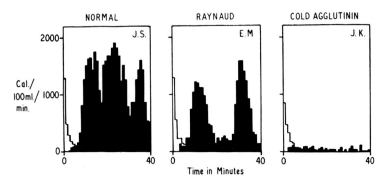

Fig. 1–8. Cooling of the fingertip of a normal subject, a patient with primary Raynaud's disease, and a patient with cold agglutinins in 0–2°C water. The clear areas represent heat derived from the tissues of the finger when cooling to calorimeter temperature during the first few minutes of immersion; the black areas represent the heat loss from the circulating blood. Cooling markedly decreases blood flow (calorimetry), but then the heat elimination of the finger rises. The blood flow of the finger fluctuates slowly, with periods of vasoconstriction alternating with vasodilatation. A similar response occurs in the finger of a patient with Raynaud's phenomenon, but the vasodilatation periods are not seen in a patient with vasospastic attacks due to cold agglutinins. *Source:* Marshall et al., 1953. Reprinted by permission from *Clinical Science* 12: 255–63 © 1953. The Biochemical Society, London.

calf, or dorsum of the hand or foot. The A-V anastomoses have been directly observed to dilate in the cold in the rabbit's ear and the bird's foot (Grant, 1930; Grant and Bland, 1931).

The mechanism of this cold vasodilatation is unknown. It is present after interruption of the sympathetic nerves by local anesthesia or chronic denervation. However, there is an influence of the sympathetic nervous system, as cold exposure of the body delays and attenuates the vasodilatory response (Keating, 1957). It is not a local axon reflex, as it is present in a fingertip locally injected with anesthetic solution (Greenfield et al., 1952). Atropine and antihistamines do not affect the response (Whittow, 1955).

This cold-induced vasodilatation serves to warm the exposed extremities sufficiently to preserve movement and sensation. However, it occurs at the cost of a considerable loss of body heat. The loss of heat from one hand (800 calories per minute in a warm person) can cause a fall in esophageal temperature of 0.6°C in 9 minutes (Greenfield et al., 1950).

Young adults and men have the greatest cold vasodilatory response (Yoshimura and Iida, 1952). Racial differences have been shown in that Blacks have less cold vasodilatation and Japanese have a greater response than Caucasians (Hirai et al., 1970; Iampietro et al., 1959). These and other studies indicate that the cold vasodilatation reaction may determine the sensitivity of a group or race to cold (Krog et al., 1960).

MECHANISMS OF DIGITAL VASODILATION

β-Adrenoceptors

Intraarterial isoproterenol causes vasodilation in the forearm but only slight or transient effects in the hand or foot. However, when the digital vascular bed was constricted with an intraarterial infusion of norepinephrine, isoproterenol (0.025–0.1 μg/min) increased total finger blood flow from 13.0 ± 5.9 to 37.0 ± 7.5 ml·min^{-1} 100 ml^{-1} of tissue (Cohen and Coffman, 1981) (Fig. 1–9). Infusion of propranolol (0.5 mg) to block the β-adrenoceptors inhibited the effect of isoproterenol. It also potentiated the vasoconstriction caused by norepinephrine, indicating that norepinephrine stimulates β-adrenoceptors as well as α-adrenoceptors.

Isoproterenol was also shown to cause vasodilation during vasoconstriction induced by intraarterial infusion of angiotensin. During the vasodilation produced by isoproterenol, capillary blood flow was unchanged. During reflex sympathetic vasoconstriction induced by body cooling, isoproterenol did not attenuate and propranolol did not potentiate the digital vasoconstriction. Also, the finger vasoconstriction produced by tyramine, which releases norepinephrine from sympathetic nerve endings, was not affected by isoproterenol. Thus there is a β-adrenergic vasodilator mechanism in human digital A-V shunts that may be humorally activated but that has no apparent functional role in modulating sympathetic vasoconstriction.

Fig. 1–9. Fingertip vascular resistance (total finger blood flow measured by plethysmography divided by the mean systemic blood pressure) shows a significant increase during intraarterial (IA) infusion of norepinephrine (NE). Isoproterenol (ISO) added to the infusion then decreased vascular resistance, indicating the presence of β-adrenoceptors. Also, propranolol (PROP), a β-adrenoceptor antagonist, added to a norepinephrine infusion potentiated the increase in vascular resistance, indicating that norepinephrine was stimulating β-adrenoceptors. *Source:* Cohen and Coffman (1981).

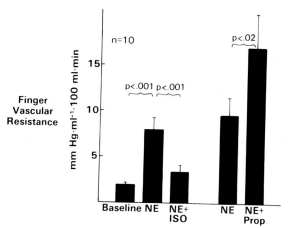

Histaminergic Receptors

There are at least two receptors (H_1 and H_2) whose stimulation may cause vasodilation in animal and human vascular beds. In cooled normal subjects, intraarterial histamine (0.5–4.0 μg/min) infusions increased total finger blood flow from 15.3 to 28.3 ml$\cdot$min^{-1} 100 ml^{-1} of tissue (Coffman et al., 1984). Finger capillary flow also increased. A-V shunt flow was probably affected, as increases in total finger blood flow were sometimes large. Neither cimetidine (H_2 selective antagonist) or pyrilamine (H_1 selective antagonist) prevented the histamine-induced increase in finger blood flow, although administration of the two antihistamines together attenuated the response. Histamine was also shown to cause a large increase in finger blood flow during vasoconstriction caused by intraarterial norepinephrine. Thus histamine can vasodilate fingertips and increase capillary and A-V blood flow during reflex sympathetic vasoconstriction caused by body cooling and during norepinephrine-induced vasoconstriction. The vasodilation may be mediated by both H_1 and H_2 receptors. The physiological importance of the digital histaminergic receptor remains to be determined.

Cholinergic Vasodilator Mechanism

Methacholine (10–80 μg/min), given by intraarterial infusion, did not affect total finger blood flow or vascular resistance in normal subjects (Coffman and Cohen, 1987). However, finger capillary blood flow showed a large, significant increase. Atropine (0.2 mg) has no effect on finger flow but inhibited the increase in capillary flow caused by methacholine. It is of interest that cholinesterase is present in the A-V anastomoses of human digital skin, as shown by histochemical techniques (Hurley and Mescon, 1956); the methacholine may therefore be metabolized before it acts on shunt vasculature. Thus a muscarinic cholinergic vasodilator mechanism exists in the fingertip that primarily affects capillary blood flow. Cholinergic agents could dilate finger blood vessels by inhibiting the release of norepinephrine from sympathetic vasoconstrictor nerves or by an indirect action on endothelial cells. A physiological role for this cholinergic mechanism has not been determined.

Neurogenic Vasodilatation

Lewis and Pickering (1931) presented evidence for sympathetic vasodilator nerves in patients with primary Raynaud's disease. In the cold-exposed fingers, the temperature of the fifth finger usually could not be increased by anesthetizing the ulnar nerve, whereas body warming produced an increase. These authors attempted to demonstrate this response in the ear and paw of the cat and obtained variable results; vasodilator sympathetic action was not found in normal men. Blumberg and Wallin (1987) have clearly demonstrated the existence of neurally mediated vasodilatation in the hairy skin of the human foot by intraneural stimulation of the superficial peroneal nerve at the ankle in normal subjects. This painful unilateral stimulation produced vasodilatation (laser–doppler flowmeters, photoelectrical pulse plethysmography) in both feet that was blocked by proximal local anesthesia of the nerve. At the same time, there was vasoconstriction of the fingers. The reflex vasodilatation of the opposite foot was enhanced by body cooling and unaffected by atropine or propranolol. With local anesthesia of the nerve, increased stimulation strength could produce localized vasodilatation in the foot that also was not blocked by atropine or propranolol. It was inhibited by capsaicin, suggesting a peptide as the neurotransmitter.

Local Axon Reflex

Stimulation of peripheral cutaneous pain nerves or other afferent nerves causes local vasodilatation. It occurs via a local axon reflex, with fibers from these nerves also innervating local blood vessels; the response can be blocked by a local nerve block.

TECHNIQUES TO MEASURE FINGER BLOOD FLOW

In order to evaluate research investigations concerning the pathogenesis and treatment of Raynaud's phenomenon, the physician must be able to evaluate the techniques to measure finger blood flow. Quantitative techniques to measure total finger blood flow include venous occlusion plethysmography and calorimetry. Qualitative methods that estimate changes in total finger blood flow are skin temperature measurements and photoplethysmography. Laser–doppler techniques have been used to measure local areas of blood flow. Capillary blood flow can be estimated by the disappearance rate of a radioisotope from the fingertip.

Venous Occlusion Plethysmography

A finger cup with a small tubular outlet usually serves as the plethysmograph and encloses the terminal phalanx of the finger (Fig. 1–10). The opening is sealed with caulking compound to make it air-tight. Stiff plastic or rubber tubing connects the tubular outlet to a sensitive pressure transducer to measure changes in fingertip volume on a recorder. A small blood pressure cuff is placed proximal to the finger cup to produce venous occlusion; a 24-mm bladder gives the most exact measurements of systolic blood pressure, so it can be used for both measurements (Gundersen, 1973; Hirai et al., 1976). During venous occlusion the fingertip swells proportional to arterial inflow for several pulse beats (Fig. 1–11). The venous occlusion pressure that produces the fastest increase in finger volume with time must be determined for each subject; it usually is 50 to 80 mm Hg. The tangent of the angle is measured for the increase in finger volume with time, multiplied by the speed of the recording paper, and divided by the calibration factor to obtain the blood flow. The system can be calibrated by introducing known quantities of air. To convert blood flow to milliliters per 100 ml of tissue, the volume of the finger in the plethysmograph can be measured by water displacement. The final formula to convert increase in volume with time to blood flow is as follows.

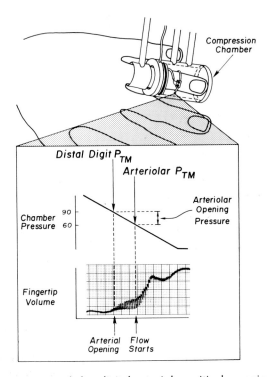

Fig. 1–10. Measurement of the digital arteriolar critical opening pressure using a compression chamber and a strain gauge on the fingertip. The chamber pressure is increased to suprasystolic pressure, which obliterates the finger pulses detected by the strain gauge. As the compression chamber pressure is slowly released to 90 mm Hg, arterial pulsations reappear without a change in finger volume (distal digital P_{TM}) indicating that the digital arteries are open. On further decompression of the chamber to 60 mm Hg, the volume of the finger increases as blood flow resumes (arteriolar P_{TM}). The critical opening pressure of the arterioles is the pressure at the reappearance of blood flow (arteriolar P_{TM}) subtracted from the pressure at which the digital arteries reopened (distal digital P_{TM}). *Source: Cohen RA, Coffman JD (1989).*

$$\frac{\text{Speed of recording paper (mm/min)}}{\text{Calibration factor (mm/1 ml)}} \times \text{tangent angle} \times \frac{100}{\text{volume of finger}}$$

Venous occlusion plethysmography has been determined to be exact if the angle of the blood flows can be kept between 30 and 60 degrees. The method is inadequate for high blood flows, as the finger fills so quickly the error of estimating the tangent of the angle is great; furthermore, for large angles, small changes yield large changes in calculated flow. Conversely, in fingers with fibrosed subcutaneous tissue, as in patients with sclerodactyly, there is little vascular space to fill during venous occlusion, and flows are difficult to measure. Mercury-in-Silastic strain gauges may be used instead of finger cups if they can be calibrated (Fig. 1–10). The circumference of the finger must then be measured. The formula for blood flow is the following.

$$\frac{\text{Speed of recording paper (mm/min)} \times 100 \times 2}{\text{Calibration for 1 mm} \times \text{circumference of finger (mm)}} \times \text{tangent angle}$$

Radioisotope Disappearance Rates

The inert gas xenon 133 can be injected or applied over the skin by various enclosure devices, after which its clearance is measured by external counting. The technique yields a clearance curve of two (Sejrsen, 1968) or three (Fares et al., 1976) components that are postulated to represent back-diffusion of the radioisotope into the atmosphere, dermal capillary blood flow, and subcutaneous blood flow. $Na^{131}I$ can be used in a similar manner but is not as freely diffusible as xenon 133 and may not follow high flow rates. Absolute flow values can be estimated by dividing the half-time of the disappearance rate by the logarithm of 2 and multiplying by the tissue coefficient of the isotope. The disappearance rates are assumed to represent capillary blood flow and correlate well with venous occlusion plethysmography in areas devoid of arteriovenous anastomoses (Walder, 1955).

Laser–Doppler Flowmeter

A laser–doppler flowmeter delivers a monochromatic light from a laser via an optical fiber. The broadening of the back-scattered laser light that results from the doppler shift produced by the reflected light from moving cells, mostly erythrocytes, in the tissue can be converted to a qualitative blood flow measurement. The broad spectrum of frequencies of reflected light is due to the different velocities of the moving cells and the fact that the laser beam hits these cells at varying angles. The laser–doppler measurements have been shown to be proportional to the product of the number of erythrocytes moving in the lighted area and the average velocity of the cells in vitro systems. Smits and co-workers (1986) compared this method with electromagnetic flowmeter or radioactive microsphere measurements of blood flow in the rat renal cortex, gracilis muscle, and cremaster muscle. The laser–doppler individual readings were variable, but mean readings from multiple areas on the

Fig. 1–11. Finger plethysmographic tracings during norepinephrine and isoproterenol infusions. During venous occlusion by a small blood pressure cuff proximal to a finger cup, the volume of the fingertip increases proportional to arterial inflow. The baseline blood flow is large, and the fingertip fills quickly. During vasoconstriction induced by intraarterial norepinephrine, the fingertip volume increases at a slower rate.

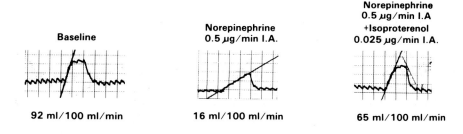

Baseline	Norepinephrine 0.5 μg/min I.A.	Norepinephrine 0.5 μg/min I.A +Isoproterenol 0.025 μg/min I.A.
92 ml/100 ml/min	16 ml/100 ml/min	65 ml/100 ml/min

tissues significantly correlated with tissue blood flow. However, significant differences in the laser–doppler flowmeter signal, compared with results of other methods, have been observed in different tissues and with different methods of measurement in the same tissue. Therefore the instrument would have to be calibrated for each use if quantitative data are to be obtained. Engelhart and Kristensen (1983) compared the laser–doppler flowmeter with the epicutaneous xenon 133 application technique. Hand cutaneous blood flow results were comparable with results obtained by the two techniques, but the calculated fingertip blood flow was fivefold larger by the laser–doppler technique. The authors therefore surmised, because xenon 133 flow was similar for the hand and finger, that the laser–doppler was measuring both capillary and A-V shunt flow.

There are several drawbacks to the use of the laser–doppler method to measure cutaneous blood flow. The depth of penetration of the laser light is unknown but is probably about 1 mm (Oberg et al., 1984). Because it is sensitive to changes in the vascular bed geometry and optical properties of the tissue, another method of flow measurement should be used for calibration. During an arterial occlusion, the flowmeter does not read zero owing to movements of muscle cells, vessel walls, various membranes, and possibly small to-and-fro movements of red blood cells. These factors can introduce errors of 8 percent in the fingertip to 15 percent in the skinfold beween fingers (Engelhart and Kristensen, 1983). Finally, the method may be more sensitive to increases in blood flow than to vasoconstriction (Sundberg and Castren, 1986); hand cutaneous blood flow decreased only 20 percent after a 5-minute exposure to frozen cold packs. Also, Kastrup and co-workers (1987) found that the laser–doppler and xenon 133 methods were not comparable; the laser–doppler method did not follow blood flow changes induced by local sympathetic-mediated venoarteriolar vasoconstriction induced by lowering the human leg below heart level. Therefore until the accuracy of the laser–doppler method is better documented, it should not be used alone in studies of the cutaneous blood flow in man.

Calorimetry

With calorimetry, quantitative estimations of heat elimination from a given volume of finger are measured and converted to blood flow. Heat elimination may be measured by a thermometer or heat flow discs stuck to the pulp of a terminal phalange placed in a calorimeter with water maintained at 29°C and vigorously stirred (Greenfield and Shepherd, 1950). Because cold blood returning from the immersed fingertip may cool arriving arterial blood, the arms are wrapped in electrically heated cloth to prevent precooling of arterial blood arriving at the digits. Measurement of the heat dissipated from the fingers correlates well with total finger blood flow measured by plethysmography. This method is difficult to use correctly and is therefore employed infrequently.

Skin Temperatures

Skin temperature is often used as an indication of finger blood flow. In a constant-temperature environment, skin temperature is linearly related to blood flow but not at low or high skin temperatures. Blood flow may increase little in a cold finger, although skin temperature rises disproportionately; in warm fingers, blood flow may increase much more than skin temperature.

FINGERTIP VASCULAR RESISTANCE

Because finger blood flow may vary with increases or decreases in perfusion pressure, changes in the blood vessels of vasodilation or vasoconstriction cannot be predicted from measurements of only finger blood flow. It is usual practice to calculate vascular resistance in order to take into account changes in blood pressure. Vascular resistance can be calculated by dividing the mean blood pressure of the digit by the digital blood flow. However, there is no method to measure digital mean blood pressure exactly. Systolic blood pressure of the finger can be determined, but diastolic pressure can be only estimated. The methods used to estimate digital diastolic or mean blood pressure have been compared to those used to determine brachial artery pressure (Kato et al., 1977; Yamakoshi et al., 1982), although they may not be the same under all circumstances. For instance, during vasodilation of the fingers produced by local warming, the digital blood pressure is less than the brachial artery blood pressure. However, the brachial artery mean pressure has been used in the resistance formula and is probably as good an estimation as can now be obtained. Digital vascular resistance, of course, shows the same wide range of variability as digital blood flow.

DIGITAL CRITICAL CLOSING OR OPENING PRESSURE

The digital critical closing (CCP) and digital critical opening (COP) pressures are indexes of vascular tone, the constricting force exerted by the vascular smooth muscle in the wall of small blood vessels. According to Burton (1951), they are expressed in terms of the transmural pressure required to close vessels from their unstretched radius (CCP) or to open vessels to their unstretched radius (COP). Some investigators have considered these determinations a better direct measurement of vascular smooth muscle reactivity or vascular tone than the indirect calculation of vascular resistance. Usually a change in CCP or COP is accompanied by an inverse change in blood flow and a parallel change in vascular resistance. It is not always the case, however. CCP and COP are regarded as indicating activity of the arterioles, but other vessels, e.g., metarterioles and precapillary sphincters, may have critical closing pressures. It is important to remember that the CCP or COP measurement is only of the vessels with the lowest CCP or COP. In the digits, the CCP or COP measures the activity of two vascular beds: the A-V shunts and the capillaries. These beds may be affected separately by stimuli and might cause the CCP or COP to be affected differently than the vascular resistance, as small changes may occur in the critical pressures, with larger changes in vascular resistance, with dilation of the shunts.

The CCP is measured by applying external pressure on the distal digit during measurement of an index of digital blood flow. The pressure at which blood flow stops is subtracted from the digital systolic blood pressure (the point of disappearance of arterial pulsations) to give the CCP. To measure COP, the pressure is increased above systolic blood pressure so that digital blood flow and pulsations stop, and then is slowly released. The pressure at the reappearance of blood flow subtracted from the pressure where fingertip pulsations first appeared, the digital systolic pressure, is the COP (Fig. 1–10). A variety of measures to detect the disappearance or reappearance of blood flow in the finger have been used, e.g., heat flow disks, microscopic observation of nailfold capillaries, spectroscopy of oxyhemoglobin absorption bands, and various plethysmography techniques. The CCP and COP are of the same order of magnitude (Gaskell, 1965; Roddie and Shepherd, 1957).

In young female subjects in a relaxed state or with digital nerve block, the COP varies from 2 to 19 mm Hg (Gaskell, 1965). However, usually after digital nerve blocks or body heating to inhibit the sympathetic nerves, the COP decreases.

Cohen and Coffman (unpublished observations) measured the COP in human fingertips by changing the external pressure within a fingertip chamber to vary transmural pressure; a strain gauge was used to detect blood flow. They found that

Fig. 1–12. Critical opening pressure (AOP) and blood flow were measured during the reflex sympathetic stimulation of environmental cooling (white bars and cross-hatched bars). Following digital nerve anesthesia to block the sympathetic nerves, the AOP decreased and fingertip blood flow increased (black bars) in both normal subjects and patients with primary Raynaud's disease. These experiments demonstrated that sympathetic nerve activity increases AOP and decreases fingertip blood flow. *Source:* Cohen RA, Coffman JD (1989).

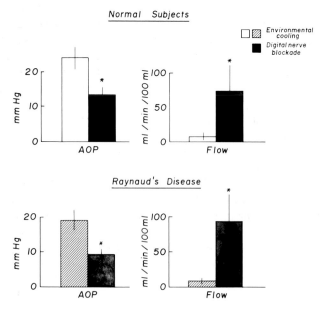

sympathetic nerve activity increased the COP during environmental cooling (20°C), as demonstrated by a decrease in COP following digital nerve blockade in both normal subjects and patients with Raynaud's disease (Fig. 1–12). Local cooling (20°C) of the nerve-blocked digit also increased the COP. The increases in COP due to the two cooling stimuli were associated with decreases in finger blood flow; however, the measure of vascular tone was different from that of vascular resistance, as greatly different reductions in blood flow and increases in vascular resistance were accompanied by equal increases of tone. These studies demonstrate that sympathetic nerve activity influences vascular smooth muscle of the small digital vessels (vascular resistance) to a greater extent than that of digital arteries (COP). Also, the increase in COP and fall in fingertip blood flow in the nerve-blocked finger indicate that local cooling increases small vessel digital vascular tone independently of sympathetic nerve activity.

Intravenous norepinephrine (5 μg/min) has been shown to increase the COP in both warm and cool fingers, but the larger increase occurred in warm fingers (Gaskell and Hoeppner, 1967). Intravenous epinephrine and vasopressin have also been shown to increase the finger COP (Gaskell, 1973). However, angiotensin II at 2 to 16 mμg/kg/min decreased the COP, whereas total digital vascular resistance was increased, as measured by venous occlusion plethysmography (Gaskell, 1967). Thus angiotensin decreased digital vascular tone but increased vascular resistance. This difference is postulated to be related to some segments of the arterial tree contracting while others relax; i.e., relaxation of arterioles would lower COP, but closure of many precapillary sphincters could raise vascular resistance.

SUMMARY

The vascular bed of the fingers consists of a capillary network for nutritional blood flow and a large number of A-V anastomoses important for the control of body and digit temperature. Total fingertip blood flow is best measured by venous occlusion plethysmography or calorimetry, and capillary blood flow is measured by the disappearance rate of radioisotopes from local application or injection. Qualitative estimates of total finger flow can be made with skin temperature measurements or laser–doppler flowmeters. Measurement of the critical opening or closing pressure yields an index of digital vascular tone. Finger blood flow is mainly under the control of the sympathetic nervous system, vasodilatation occurring by withdrawal of activity and vasoconstriction by stimulation. An active vasodilatory neurogenic mechanism in the fingers has not been found. The sympathetic activity is modulated by the cerebral cortex, hypothalamus, medullary vasomotor centers, and spinal cord. Reflex sympathetic vasoconstriction is mediated mainly through the α_2-adrenoceptors, which predominantly affect the A-V anastomoses. Local cooling induces fingertip vasoconstriction but at a temperature of less than 10°C, periods of vasodilatation alternate with periods of vasoconstriction. This process is evidently a protective mechanism that preserves finger movement and sensation. S_2-serotonergic receptors are present in the digital vasculature and affect both capillary and A-V shunt blood flow. They are involved in the vasoconstriction seen during reflex sympathetic stimulation by body cooling. β-Adrenoceptors are present in the A-V anastomoses but evidently react only to circulating catecholamines and not sympathetic nerve activity. Histaminergic and cholinergic receptors have also been demonstrated, but their physiological importance is unknown. The cholinergic mechanism is especially interesting, as only capillary blood flow is affected.

REFERENCES

Arneklo-Nobin B, Owman C: Adrenergic and serotonergic mechanisms in human hand arteries and veins studied by fluorescence histochemistry and in vitro pharmacology. *Blood Vessels* 22:1, 1985.

Blumberg H, Wallin GB: Direct evidence of neurally mediated vasodilatation in hairy skin of the human foot. *J Physiol* (Lond) 382:105, 1987.

Burton, AC: On the physical equilibrium of small blood vessels. *Am J Physiol* 164:319, 1951.

Burton, AC, Taylor RM: A study of the adjustment of peripheral vascular tone to the requirements of the regulation of body temperature. *Am J Physiol* 129:565, 1940.

Coffman JD: Total and nutritional blood flow in the finger. *Clin Sci* 42:243, 1972.

Coffman JD, Cohen RA: A cholinergic vasodilator mechanism in the human finger. *Am J Physiol* 252:H594, 1987.

Coffman JD, Cohen RA: Role of alpha-adrenoceptor subtypes mediating sympathetic vasoconstriction in human digits. *Eur J Clin Invest* 18:390, 1988a.

Coffman JD, Cohen RA: Serotonergic vasoconstriction in human fingers during reflex sympathetic response to cooling. *Am J Physiol* 254:H889, 1988b.

Coffman JD, Cohen RA: α-Adrenergic and serotonergic mechanisms in the human digit. *J Cardiovasc Pharmacol* II (Supp 1); S49, 1988c.

Coffman JD, Cohen RA, Rasmussen HM: The effect of histamine on human fingertip circulation. *Clin Sci* 66:343, 1984.

Cohen RA, Coffman JD: β-Adrenergic vasodilator mechanism in the finger. *Circ Res* 49:1196, 1981.

Cohen RA, Coffman JD: Reduced fingertip arterial pressures in Raynaud's disease. *J Vasc Med Biol* 1:21, 1989.

Coleman SS, Anson BJ: Arterial patterns in the hand based upon a study of 650 specimens. *Surg Gynecol Obstet* 113:409, 1961.

Doscher W, Viswanathan B, Stein T, Margolis IB: Hemodynamic assessment of the circulation in 200 normal hands. *Ann Surg* 198:776, 1983.

Engelhart M, Kristensen JK: Evaluation of cutaneous blood flow responses by [133]xenon washout and a laser–doppler flowmeter. *J Invest Dermatol* 80:12, 1983.

Engelhart M, Kristensen JK: Raynaud's phenomenon: blood supply to fingers during indirect cooling, evaluated by laser doppler flowmetry. *Clin Physiol* 6:481, 1986.

Fares CM, Milliken JC, Beckett VL: Digital skin capillary flow of xenon-133 in rheumatoid arthritis. *Ir J Med Sci* 145:217, 1976.

Flavahan NA, Cooke JP, Shepherd JT, Vanhoutte PM: Human postjunctional alpha-1 and alpha-2 adrenoceptors: differential distribution in arteries of the limbs. *J Pharmacol Exp Ther* 241:361, 1987.

Gaskell P: The measurement of blood pressure, the critical opening pressure, and the critical closing pressure of digital vessels under various circumstances. *Can J Physiol Pharmacol* 43:979, 1965.

Gaskell P: Digital vascular response to angiotensin II in normotensive and hypertensive subjects. *Circ Res* 20:174, 1967.

Gaskell P: The influence of lysine-8-vasopressin, oxytocin, and adrenaline on vascular smooth muscle in the human finger. *Can J Physiol Pharmacol* 51:284, 1973.

Gaskell P, Hoeppner DL: The effect of local temperature on the reactivity to noradrenaline of digital vessels. *Can J Physiol Pharmacol* 45:93, 1967.

Grant RT: Observations on direct communications between arteries and veins in the rabbit's ear. *Heart* 15:281, 1930.

Grant RT, Bland EF: Observations on arteriovenous anastomoses in human skin and in the bird's foot with special reference to the reaction to cold. *Heart* 15:385, 1931.

Greenfield ADM, Shepherd JT: A quantitative study of the response to cold of the circulation through the fingers of normal subjects. *Clin Sci* 9:323, 1950.

Greenfield ADM, Shepherd JT, Whelan RF: The loss of heat from the hands and from the fingers immersed in cold water. *J Physiol* (Lond) 112:459, 1950.

Greenfield ADM, Shepherd JT, Whelan RF: Circulatory response to cold in fingers infiltrated with anesthetic solution. *J Appl Physiol* 4:785, 1952.

Griffith SG, Lincoln J, Burnstock G: Serotonin as a neurotransmitter in cerebral arteries. *Brain Res* 247:388, 1982.

Gundersen J: Measurement of systolic blood pressure in all fingers. *Dan Med Bull* 20:129, 1973.

Hirai K, Horvath, SM, Weinstein V: Differences in the vascular hunting reaction between Caucasians and Japanese. *Angiology* 21:502, 1970.

Hirai M, Nielsen SL, Lassen NA: Blood pressure measurement of all five fingers by strain gauge plethysmography. *Scand J Clin Lab Invest* 36:627, 1976.

Hurley HJ, Mescon H: Cholinergic innervation of the digital arterio-venous anastomoses of human skin: a histochemical localization of cholinesterase. *J Appl Physiol* 9:82, 1956.

Iampietro PF, Goldman RF, Buskirk ER, Bass DE: Response of Negro and white males to cold. *J Appl Physiol* 14:798, 1959.

Jauernig RA, Moulds RFW, Shaw J: The action of prazosin in human vascular preparations. *Arch Int Pharmacodyn* 231:81, 1978.

Kastrup J, Bulow J, Lassen NA: A comparison between [133]xenon washout technique and laser doppler flowmetry in the measurement of local vasoconstrictor effects on the microcirculation in subcutaneous tissue and skin. *Clin Physiol* 7:403, 1987.

Kato M, Toshihko K, Inomata H, Motoyama A, Nakai K, Kimura T, Chiba T: Measurement of digital arterial blood pressure and its recording on usual electrocardiograph paper. *Tohoku J Exp Med* 123:307, 1977.

Keating WR: Effect of general chilling on the vasodilator response to cold. *J Physiol* (Lond) 139;497, 1957.

Keen JA: A study of the arterial variations in the limbs, with special reference to symmetry of vascular patterns. *Am J Anat* 108:245, 1961.

Kitamura K, Hangyo K, Yamaji K: Finger blood flow decrease in leg exercise. *Jpn J Physiol* 32:141, 1982.

Kristensen JK, Engelhart, M, Nielsen T: Laser-doppler measurement of digital blood flow regulation in normals and in patients with Raynaud's phenomenon. *Acta Derm Venereol* (Stockh) 63:43, 1983.

Krog J, Folkow B, Fox RH, Andersen KL: Hand circulation in the cold of Lapps and North Norwegian fishermen. *J Appl Physiol* 15:654, 1960.

Lewis T: Observations upon reactions of vessels of human skin to cold. *Heart* 15:177, 1930.

Lewis T, Pickering GW: Vasodilatation in the limbs in response to warming the body; with evidence for sympathetic vasodilator nerves in man. *Heart* 16:34, 1931.

Little JM, Zylstra PL, West J, May J: Circulatory patterns in the normal hand. *Brt J Surg* 60:652, 1973.

Marshall RJ, Shepherd JT, Thompson ID: Vascular responses in patients with high serum titres of cold agglutinins. *Clin Sci* 12:255, 1953.

Nagasaka T, Cabanac M, Hirata K, Nunomura T: Heat-induced vasoconstriction in the fingers: a mechanism for reducing heat gain through the hand heated locally. *Pflugers Arch* 407:71, 1986.

Oberg PA, Tenland T, Nilsson GE: Laser-doppler flowmetry: a non-invasive and continuous method for blood flow evaluation in microvascular studies. *Acta Med Scand* [Suppl] 687:17, 1984.

Prichard MML, Daniel PM: Arteriovenous anastomoses in the human external ear. *J Anat* 90:309, 1956.

Roddie LC, Shepherd JT: Evidence for critical closure of digital resistance vessels with reduced transmural pressure and passive dilatation with increased venous pressure. *J Physiol* (Lond) 136:498, 1957.

Roddie LC, Shepherd JT, Whelan RF: The action of 5-hydroxytryptamine on the blood vessels of the human hand and forearm. *Brt J Pharmacol Chemother* 10:445, 1955.

Rowell LB, Brengelmann GL, Detry J-MR, Wyss C: Venomotor responses to rapid changes in skin temperature in exercising man. *J Appl Physiol* 30:64, 1971.

Sejrsen P: Atraumatic local labelling of skin by inert gas: epicutaneous application of xenon-133. *J Appl Physiol* 24:570, 1968.

Smits GJ, Roman RJ, Lombard JH: Evaluation of laser-doppler flowmetry as a measure of tissue blood flow. *J Appl Physiol* 61:666, 1986.

Stevens MJ, Moulds RFW: Heterogeneity of post-junctional α-adrenoceptors in human vascular smooth muscle. *Arch Int Pharmacodyn* 254:43, 1981.

Sundberg S, Castren M: Drug- and temperature-induced changes in peripheral circulation measured by laser-doppler flowmetry and digital-pulse plethysmography. *Scand J Clin Lab Invest* 46:359, 1986.

Varro J, Lazlo H, Varga G: Anatomy of the hand arteries based on angiographic studies. *Magy Traumatol Orthop* 21:127, 1978.

Walder DN: The relationship between blood flow, capillary surface area and sodium clearance in muscle. *Clin Sci* 14:303, 1955.

Whittow GC: Effect of antihistamine substances on cold vasodilatation in the finger. *Nature* 176;511, 1955.

Yamakoshi K, Shimazu H, Shibata M, Kamiya A: New oscillometric method for indirect measurement of systolic and mean arterial pressure in the human finger. 2. Correlation study. *Med Biol Eng Comput* 20:314, 1982.

Yoshimura H, Iida T: Studies on the reactivity of skin vessels to extreme cold. *Jpn J Physiol* 1:147, 1950; 2:177, 1952; 2:310, 1952.

2

Primary Raynaud's Disease: Clinical Picture, Prevalence, and Prognosis

Maurice Raynaud's original description of Raynaud's phenomenon in 1888 has stood the test of time. He characterized the entity as occurring usually in female subjects, with the development of pale, cold, single or multiple digits brought on by the "least stimulus" or "without appreciable cause" (Fig. 2–1). The attacks of "dead fingers" varied from a few minutes to many hours. Cold was the most common precipitating cause, although sometimes a "simple mental emotion" was enough. The skin of the affected parts became dead white or sometimes yellow; numbness was a prominent feature. In rare cases the dead finger became covered with cold sweat. The toes could also be affected. In more intense cases the pallor was replaced by cyanosis. Finally, the digits turned red when recovering from the attack. The only part of Raynaud's description that turned out to be incorrect was the claim that pain was an almost constant phenomenon. With the primary disease pain is not usual during the pallor or cyanotic phase, although throbbing pain may occur during the red reactive hyperemic recovery phase.

CLINICAL PICTURE

Age

Among 474 female patients with a diagnosis of primary Raynaud's disease by Allen and Brown's criteria (see Chap. 5), the average age was 31 years (Gifford and Hines, 1957) (Table 2–1). Seventy-eight percent were 39 years of age or younger at the onset of symptoms. The oldest patient was 68. In another series of 100 patients, 60 percent had the onset of disease at age 11 to 30 years, 81 percent at 11 to 40 years. Only five patients were older than 45 years at onset (Blain et al., 1951). In a group of 100 male patients with primary Raynaud's disease, the syndrome appeared before age 40 in 73 percent; the age range was 5 to 63 years (Hines and Christensen, 1945). Abramson and Schumacher (1947) describe 50 male patients with Raynaud's phenomenon that was considered to be the primary disease; however, symp-

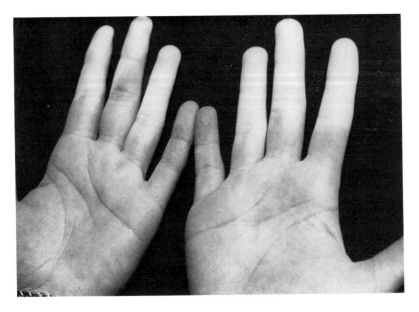

Fig. 2–1. Typical vasospastic attack in a young woman with primary Raynaud's disease. There is well demarcated pallor of the second, third, and fourth fingers that occurred during episodic attacks on exposure to cold.

toms sometimes were not present for 2 years and were often unilateral; the age range was 21 to 51 years, with an average of 29.5 years.

Sex and Race

In a series of 100 patients with primary Raynaud's disease, 77 percent were female (Blain et al., 1951); a previous study in another institution had found exactly the same female predominance (Hines and Christensen, 1945). The low incidence of the disease mandates a careful search for secondary etiologies in male patients presenting with Raynaud's phenomenon. In a prevalence study of the phenomenon (primary and secondary), Maricq and co-workers (1986) found an equal distribu-

Table 2–1. Raynaud's Phenomenon

Age of onset	11 to 45 years
Sex	77% female
Site of involvement	55–61% fingers only
	36–43% toes and fingers
Precipitating cause	Cold in 100%
	Emotions in 9 to 60%
Color changes	Triphasic 4–65%
	Biphasic 14–40%
	Only pallor or cyanosis 10–44%

tion among men and women as well as among Blacks and Whites. Four Blacks were reported in a series of 50 men with Raynaud's phenomenon (Abramson and Shumacher, 1947). Other studies of racial involvement are not available.

Symptoms

Site of Involvement

Of 474 female patients with primary Raynaud's disease, 54.6 percent had attacks only in the fingers, 42.6 percent in the fingers and toes, and less than 1 percent only in the toes. The nose, ears, face, chest, and lips were affected in some patients (Gifford and Hines, 1957). In the series of 100 patients with vasospastic attacks of the fingers (Blain and co-workers, 1951), 40 percent had involvement of the lower extremities. Of 100 male patients with primary Raynaud's disease, 61 percent had involvement of the fingers, 36 percent had attacks of both fingers and toes, and none had only the toes affected (Hines and Christensen, 1945). In this study, the attacks were unilateral in 16 percent. In the study of 50 male patients (Abramson and Shumacher, 1947), 80 percent had finger involvement, 16 percent had attacks of both fingers and toes, and 4 percent had only the toes affected; symptoms were unilateral in 12 percent.

In our experience, many patients present with only one or two fingers affected, although over the years more fingers became involved and later the toes may become symptomatic. Interestingly, the thumbs are often spared, perhaps because their digital arteries originate directly from the radial artery.

Color Phases

In the above study of primary Raynaud's disease by Gifford and Hines (1957), 65 percent of 133 patients had the classic white to blue to red digital color changes; two phases occurred in 22 percent; and one phase, usually pallor, was present in 13 percent. In the study of male patients (Hines and Christensen, 1945), the three-phase color change was present in only 22 percent of patients; pallor was the most frequent sign and occurred in 41 percent of 63 patients as the only color change. In the other male study (Abramson and Shumacher, 1947) three colors occurred in 50 percent of 50 patients, two colors in 40 percent, and one color in 10 percent.

Our patient population with the primary disease has more frequently presented with only the white color change, rather than the biphasic or triphasic picture. Maricq and co-workers (1986) also reported that white (38 percent) or blue (44 percent) color changes were more common than two (14 percent) or three (4 percent) color combinations in 78 patients with Raynaud's phenomenon (primary and secondary).

Precipitating Causes of Attacks

Cold exposure is the commonest cause of vasospastic attacks. It was the only instigating stimulus in 77 percent of 474 patients with primary Raynaud's disease (Gifford and Hines, 1957). Emotions and cold induced attacks in 18 percent. Tea or coffee was considered a factor in only one patient. In the study of 100 patients by Blain and co-workers (1951), cold exposure produced attacks in 100 percent, and emotions were said to be involved in 60 percent of patients. In some patients attacks could be caused by smoking, but in others there appeared to be no connection. In the study by Hines and Christensen (1945), of 100 male subjects with Raynaud's phenomenon there was no correlation with smoking; 9 percent reported that emotions in addition to cold exposure produced attacks. Unusual precipitating events have been attacks during the reporting of dreams in a young boy (Szajnberg et al., 1987) and during urination in a 40-year-old woman in our practice. Melmed and co-workers (1986) were able to induce vasospastic attacks by hypnotic suggestion. In our patients, cold exposure combined with pressure on the fingers, e.g., holding a steering wheel, shopping bag handle, frozen foods, or glass, is one of the most common instigating factors. Emotions may cause attacks but only in a few patients. We have been impressed with the inability to induce vasospastic attacks in the office with a combination of the instigating causes even though the patient presents with an attack.

Trophic Digital Effects

In a large study of the primary disease (Gifford and Hines, 1957), 13 percent of the women had ulcerations, chronic paronychia, necrosis, or scarring or fissuring of the fingers; sclerodactyly occurred in 12 percent. Most patients in whom we have seen these changes develop a positive antinuclear antibody test, although it may not occur until several years after the first presentation. The only clue to a secondary disease at the time of initial presentation of these patients was sometimes an elevated erythrocyte sedimentation rate.

Concomitant Diseases

In the Gifford and Hines study (1957), 9 percent of patients were hypertensive, and 14 percent had migraine headaches. Blain and co-workers (1951) mentioned that both diseases occurred in their patients but numbers were not given. Miller and co-workers (1981) reported a strong correlation of migraine headaches and variant angina pectoris in a large study of patients with Raynaud's phenomenon. If confirmed, the possibility of vasospasm occurring in three vascular beds is suggested (Coffman and Cohen, 1981) (see Chap. 4). Many of our patients have had migraine headaches, but we have not seen variant angina. The migraine headaches in these patients usually had not been treated with drugs that induce Raynaud's phenomenon.

Summary

Primary Raynaud's disease occurs in young women usually before age 45 years. Vasospastic attacks involve mainly the fingers, although they affect both fingers and toes in a large percentage of patients. Most patients' digits have been reported to undergo triphasic color changes (pallor to cyanosis to rubor), but in our experience many have only pallor. Cold combined with pressure on the digits is the most common precipitating cause; emotions induce attacks in some patients. About 13 percent of patients have trophic changes of the digits including sclerodactyly. The disease in men is similar to that in women, but more men have only pallor as a color change.

PREVALENCE

Few studies have attempted to determine the prevalence of Raynaud's phenomenon in the general population (Table 2–2). Lewis and Pickering (1934) questioned 60 men aged 20 to 45 years and 62 women aged 19 to 34 years concerning the presence of recurrent short attacks of symmetrical discoloration of the fingers and sometimes the toes during cold exposure; most subjects were medical students or nurses. Twenty-five percent of the men and 30 percent of the women said that one or more of their fingers occasionally became white or pale blue with numbness and occasional pain; redness occurred during the recovery phase.

Olsen and Nielsen (1978) determined that the frequency of Raynaud's phenomenon was 22 percent (95 percent confidence limits: 13–34 percent) in a random sample of 67 healthy female physical therapists 21 to 50 years of age in Denmark. A questionnaire was used, and Raynaud's phenomenon was defined as the appearance of white, dead fingers upon cold exposure with frequent cold or bluish fingers for more than 2 years. Local finger cooling with ischemia induced abnormal digital systolic blood pressure measurements in all eight subjects who had been tested and had been classified as having Raynaud's phenomenon according to the questionnaire. Although the investigators considered that the subjects had the primary disease, a complete work-up to exclude secondary diseases was not performed.

Heslop and co-workers (1983) surveyed 520 people aged 20 to 59 years in a general practice in Southampton, England with a questionnaire inquiring about sudden attacks of cold, numb, white fingers. Of the 450 subjects who returned the questionnaire, 50 of 73 reporting symptoms agreed to an interview, and in 40 the history was confirmed. If only the confirmed cases in the group who returned the questionnaire are considered, the minimum estimate would be that 5 percent of men and 10.4 percent of women had Raynaud's phenomenon. If the 40 confirmed cases and a similar proportion (80 percent) of the 23 subjects reporting symptoms who could not be interviewed are included, the estimate would be 8.3 percent in men and 17.6 percent in women. Unfortunately, this study did not question subjects about blue color changes.

The largest survey involved 1752 randomly selected subjects in South Carolina with a trained interviewer administering the questionnaires (Maricq et al., 1986).

Table 2–2. Prevalence of Raynaud's Phenomenon

Study	No. of pts.	Sex	Age (years)	Etiology	Raynaud's phenomenon (%)
Lewis & Pickering (1934)	60	M	20–45	Primary?	25
	62	F	19–34	Primary?	30
Olsen & Nielsen (1978)	67	F	21–50	Primary?	22
Heslop et al. (1983)[a]	520	MF	20–59	Unknown	5.0–8.3 M 10.4–17.6F
Maricq et al. (1986)	1752	MF	> 18	Unknown	4.6

[a]Questionnaire included only white, not blue, fingers.

Their estimate of the prevalence of Raynaud's phenomenon, if only cold-sensitive subjects reporting white or blue digital color changes were included, was 4.6 percent. The subjects in this study were of both sexes and over 18 years of age. Some subjects selected by the questionnaire may have had secondary diseases because complaints of swollen fingers and dysphagia were common, as was the use of vibratory tools. Other studies have mentioned the prevalence of Raynaud's phenomenon in patients with other diseases such as hypertension, and some surveys did not adequately define the syndrome.

In summary, studies show a prevalence of Raynaud's phenomenon in 4.6 to 30.0 percent of randomly questioned people. The largest survey favors the lower percentage, but that survey was conducted using people in a warmer climate than the other studies. There is no information available concerning the prevalence of Raynaud's phenomenon in different temperature zones. Although it is probable that the available studies included more patients with the primary disease, this prevalence is by no means certain, and therefore the prevalence of primary versus secondary Raynaud's phenomenon in a general population remains unknown. Prevalence studies are needed in different climates and with documentation of the primary or secondary etiology of the disease.

PROGNOSIS

Gifford and Hines (1957) were able to obtain follow-up information on 307 of 397 patients with Raynaud's phenomenon presumably primary in nature. These patients had received only medical treatment, if any, for an average of 12 years. They had had symptoms for 3 to 46 years, with an average duration of 17 years. Thirty-eight percent reported no change in symptoms, 36 percent improved, 16 percent were worse, and the syndrome disappeared in 10 percent. Sclerodactyly disappeared in 19 of 27 patients and was unchanged in 7 patients; it developed in 3.3 percent. Calcinosis was present in 1.3 percent (four patients). Only 0.4 percent (two patients) had digital amputations for ulcers, although 13 percent had ulceration, chronic paronychia, necrosis of skin, scarring, or fissuring. Tobacco smoking did not seem to affect the prognosis. Of the 44 patients who moved to a warmer climate, symptoms were alleviated in just over one-half. None of the patients with the onset of symptoms before 10 or after 55 years of age had serious or disabling conditions. One problem with this study is that the more severely afflicted patients were eliminated because they underwent surgery. It was also before the time of the more sophisticated tests that are now available for diagnosing connective tissue diseases. Blain and co-workers (1951), who included both medically and surgically treated patients in their study of primary Raynaud's disease, reported that 48 percent of patients noted slight to severe progression of symptoms, 40 percent remained unchanged, and 12 percent had regression or disappearance of the syndrome.

In a more recent study, Clavijo and Krahenbuhl (1981) followed 136 patients with primary or secondary Raynaud's phenomenon for an average of 3.9 years.

Improvement occurred in 36 percent, there was no change in 48 percent, and deterioration was seen in 16 percent. These figures agree remarkably well with the Gifford and Hines study of patients with primary Raynaud's disease. Of the 25 patients with the primary disease, 25 percent improved and 12 percent worsened. Clavijo and Krahenbuhl concluded that a combination of an abnormal Allen's test, digital skin necrosis, age greater than 60 years, and a history of vasospastic attacks for more than 1 year predicted a poor prognosis.

The presence of Raynaud's phenomenon and sclerodactyly evidently does not predict a dire prognosis. Farmer and colleagues (1961) followed 71 patients with sclerodactyly and a diagnosis of primary Raynaud's disease by the Allen and Brown criteria for an average of 10 years (2–31 years). Forty were treated medically, and 31 underwent sympathectomy. Twenty-six had trophic changes of ulcers, fissures, or chronic paronychia. The outcome was similar despite treatment; 20 patients improved, 16 deteriorated, 29 were unchanged, and 6 died of unrelated causes (three treated medically and three surgically). Three medical and five surgical patients developed trophic changes during follow-up, although scleroderma developed in only three patients (4 percent). Although trophic changes of the fingers are present or develop in many patients with sclerodactyly, the prognosis is fairly good.

Gerbracht and co-workers (1985) studied the evolution of primary Raynaud's disease to connective tissue disease. Eighty-seven patients initially diagnosed as having the primary disease had vasospastic attacks for at least 2 years and were followed an average of 5.1 years (2.8–9.1 years) after the onset of symptoms. Four of 87 patients (5 percent) ultimately developed a connective tissue disease, and each had scleroderma of the CREST variety (see Chap. 6). Other patients could develop connective tissue diseases later, as 17 percent of patients had antinuclear antibodies; however, the authors concluded that connective tissue disease infrequently develops during the ensuing decade in patients considered to have primary Raynaud's disease except for laboratory and serological abnormalities. Similarly, Harper and co-workers (1982) found that 3 of 39 patients (8 percent), whose only clinical manifestation was Raynaud's phenomenon, developed a connective tissue disease after a mean follow-up period of 2 years but a duration of vasospastic attacks of 7 years. Both of these studies included patients in the category of only Raynaud's phenomenon even when abnormal laboratory studies were present.

Classifying patients on the basis of history, physical examination, hand radiographs, nailfold capillary microscopy, and chest film, Priollet and colleagues (1987) followed 73 patients with Raynaud's phenomenon for an average of 4.7 years. They had vasospastic attacks for an average of 14.9 years. None of the 49 patients initially classified as having primary disease because of negative examination and tests developed evidence of a secondary etiology, whereas 14 of 24 patients with suspected secondary Raynaud's phenomenon did.

Nailfold capillary abnormalities seen by microscopy have been considered a useful prognostic indicator by some investigators. However, patients with normal capillary patterns have developed secondary diseases, and patients with abnormal patterns often do not develop connective tissue disease over short follow-up periods (Lefford and Edwards, 1986). Furthermore, a relation between capillary morphology and the clinical features of the diseases is disputed (see Chap. 5).

REFERENCES

Abramson DI, Shumacher HB Jr: Raynaud's disease in men. *Am Heart J* 33:500, 1947.

Blain A, Coller FA, Carver GB: Raynaud's disease: a study of criteria for prognosis. *Surgery* 29:387, 1951.

Clavijo F, Krahenbuhl B: Evolution naturelle du phenomene de Raynaud. *Schweiz Med Wochenschr* 111:2023, 1981.

Coffman JD, Cohen RA: Vasospasm—ubiquitous? *N Engl J Med* 304:780, 1981.

Farmer RG, Gifford RW Jr, Hines EA Jr: Raynaud's disease with sclerodactylia. *Circulation* 23:13, 1961.

Gerbracht DD, Steen VD, Ziegler GL, Medsger TA Jr, Rodnan GP: Evolution of primary Raynaud's phenomenon (Raynaud's disease) to connective tissue disease. *Arthritis Rheum* 28:87, 1985.

Gifford RW Jr, Hines EA Jr: Raynaud's disease among women and girls. *Circulation* 16:1012, 1957.

Harper FE, Maricq HR, Turner RE, Lidman RW, LeRoy EC: A prospective study of Raynaud's phenomenon and early connective tissue disease. *Am J Med* 72:883, 1982.

Heslop J, Coggon D, Acheson ED: The prevalence of intermittent digital ischaemia (Raynaud's phenomenon) in a general practice. *J Coll Gen Pract* 33:85, 1983.

Hines EA Jr, Christensen NA: Raynaud's disease affecting men. *JAMA* 129:1, 1945.

Lefford F, Edwards JC: Nailfold capillary microscopy in connective tissue disease: a quantitative morphological analysis. *Ann Rheum Dis* 45:741, 1986.

Lewis T, Pickering GW: Observations upon maladies in which the blood supply to digits ceases intermittently or permanently and upon bilateral gangrene of digits; observations relevant to so-called Raynaud's disease. *Clin Sci* 1:327, 1934.

Maricq HR, Weinrich MC, Keil JE, LeRoy EC: Prevalence of Raynaud's phenomenon in the general population. *J Chronic Dis* 39:423, 1986.

Melmed RN, Roth D, Beer G, Edelstein EL: Placebo and symptoms. *Lancet* 2:1448, 1986.

Miller D, Waters DD, Warmica W, Szlachcic J, Kreeft J, Theroux P: Is variant angina the coronary manifestation of a generalized vasospastic disorder. *N Engl J Med* 304:763, 1981.

Olsen N, Nielsen SL: Prevalence of primary Raynaud phenomena in young females. *Scand J Clin Lab Invest* 37:761, 1978.

Priollet P, Vayssairat M, Housset E: How to classify Raynaud's phenomenon. *Am J Med* 83:494, 1987.

Raynaud M: *On Local Asphyxia and Symmetrical Gangrene of the Extremities.* Translated by T. Barlow. London: The Syndenham Society, 1888, p. 99.

Szajnberg NM, Zalneraitis E, Zemel L: Unilateral Raynaud's symptoms evoked during dream report. *Lancet* 2:802, 1987.

3

Pathology and Angiography

Studies of the pathology of the digital blood vessels by histological techniques or angiography could be helpful in understanding the pathophysiology and clinical manifestations of primary or secondary Raynaud's phenomenon. This is true for some of the secondary diseases such as scleroderma, but not for the primary disease. However, lack of pathological findings does direct attention to seeking a functional mechanism of vasospasm.

PATHOLOGY

Pathology studies of the digital blood vessels in primary and secondary Raynaud's syndrome are not numerous, especially for the primary disease. Even in the few studies that have been performed, it is difficult to differentiate the lesions that may cause the syndrome from lesions caused by the ischemic episodes.

Lewis (1938) histologically examined digital arteries from two patients with mild primary Raynaud's disease and four other patients with more severe disease. The digital arteries were compared to vessels from a group of patients without Raynaud's phenomenon. In the two patients with mild disease, fewer changes were seen in the intima than in digital arteries from comparable age-matched controls. A patient with greater severity of disease showed moderate intimal hyperplasia. Hypertrophy of the media was absent. In patients with trophic lesions of the digits, intimal hyperplasia, narrowing or total occlusion of the lumen, or thrombi were present. Lewis concluded that the main pathology seen in the arterial wall in primary Raynaud's disease is hyperplasia of the intima but that this change is no greater than is seen in normal subjects. Laws and colleagues (1967), in a postmortem digital artery arteriographic and histologic study, confirmed the report of Lewis that digital arteries show increasing thickening of the intima with age in normal subjects. It is not clear if the changes observed represent early atherosclerosis, as intimal hyperplasia is a primary characteristic of that disease. In patients without Raynaud's phenomenon, complete occlusion of vessels was rare before age 50. After age 50, complete occlusion was commoner in men than women, and there was often evidence of cardiovascular disease in the coronary arteries or aorta.

Patients with rheumatoid arthritis had an increased incidence of digital vascular occlusions.

Rodnan and co-workers (1980) examined digital artery segments from 16 patients who died from scleroderma; all but one patient had Raynaud's phenomenon. The most prominent finding was severe intimal hyperplasia consisting predominantly of collagen. In most of the vessels there was severe luminal narrowing and, in some, thrombosis. Adventitial fibrosis and telangiectasia of the vasa vasorum were seen in fewer than one-half of the specimens.

Burch and co-workers (1979) studied skin specimens from punch biopsy specimens of the fingers of six patients with Raynaud's phenomenon. Four patients had scleroderma of the digits. In one patient considered to have primary Raynaud's disease, there was inflammatory destruction of the capillary bed in the superficial dermis with numerous fibroblasts replacing the capillaries. In another patient considered to have primary Raynaud's disease but with an ulcer of a finger, there was fibrinoid degeneration of the capillaries in the stratum papillare. Both patients showed segmental inflammation and edema in the walls of the small blood vessels. The other four patients with scleroderma showed a prominent diminution of capillaries and blood vessels, with extensive collagen in the dermis. The remaining capillaries had thickened walls, and some had obliterated lumens. Glomus bodies, observed in two patients, showed extensive fibrosis with thickened arterioles but open vessels. Electron microscopy of the biopsy specimens from four patients showed dissolution of the endothelial cytoplasm and desquamation of endothelial cells. The basement membranes were thickened, with incorporation of collagen fibrils. The pericytes of capillaries showed numerous rough-surfaced vesicles, many free ribosomal granules or ribonucleoprotein particles, and increased numbers of mitochrondia, suggesting increased cellular activity. Abnormalities of the glomus bodies have also been described for Raynaud's syndrome by Bauer et al. (1979).

Vajda and co-workers (1982) also studied finger pulp biopsies by light and electron microscopy from 31 patients with Raynaud's phenomenon due to a variety of underlying diseases. Two cases fitted the category of the primary disease (although one had hypertension); these patients had had vasospastic attacks for 2 to 10 years. Biopsies, from the lateral side of the distal phalanx, were compared to five normal control subjects. In the dermal capillaries, endothelium cell swelling resulted in narrowing of the lumen. There were increased numbers of intracytoplasmic filaments and Weibel-Palade bodies. The basement membranes were thickened and multilayered; occasionally a fuzzy granulomatous material replaced the basement membrane. The basement membrane of the unmyelinated nerves showed similar alterations. Severe degenerative changes were found in the myelin sheath of the myelinated axons. There was severe degeneration of the elastic fibers in the dermal connective tissue. Endothelial cell and basement membrane changes were seen in one of the two patients with primary Raynaud's disease. Because patients with recent onset of vasospastic attacks were not studied, the authors considered these findings to represent the ultrastructural picture of the end-stage of this syndrome. They considered the findings pathognomonic of the condition but not helpful for diagnosing the underlying disease causing the Raynaud's phenomenon. The study included patients with lupus erythematosus, acrocyanosis, polyarthritis, thromboangiitis obliterans, vibration-induced vasospastic disease, and other diseases, but most were scleroderma or thoracic outlet syndrome.

Thompson and co-workers (1984) performed nailfold biopsies and described a globular, eosinophilic, periodic acid-schiff (PAS)-positive material deposited in the cuticles of 14 of 15 patients with scleroderma, mixed connective tissue disease, or primary Raynaud's disease but not in the cuticles of nine controls. By immunofluorescence staining, the material proved to be a serum protein exudate; Thompson et al. hypothesized that this material resulted from increased capillary permeability. There was marked parakeratosis, and increased epithelial mitotic activity was present. They also found a decreased number of cutaneous nerve bundles in the patients. Of these 15 patients, four had Raynaud's phenomenon. Two definitely had scleroderma; two had no secondary disease, although one had scleroderma-type capillary abnormalities. Bollinger and co-workers (1986) provided further evidence of increased capillary permeability by demonstrating that the normal barriers for diffusion of fluorescein sodium from the capillaries are less effective in patients with scleroderma.

ANGIOGRAPHY

Connective Tissue Disease

Angiographic studies of scleroderma show irregular narrowing and obstruction of the digital arteries and often larger vessels in nearly all subjects with Raynaud's phenomenon (Fig. 3–1). Dabich and co-workers (1972) and Jeune and Thivolet (1978) demonstrated arterial stenosis or occlusion in the digital arteries in 28 of 31 and all of 22 patients, respectively. In the study by Dabich's group, the ulnar artery was narrowed or occluded in 16 of 31 patients and the radial artery in only two patients with scleroderma. Narrowing and obstruction of digital arteries has also been observed in patients with rheumatoid arthritis (Laws et al., 1963), systemic lupus erythematosus (Jeune and Thivolet, 1978), and polyarteritis nodosa (Laws et al., 1963). According to Laws and colleagues (1963) the occlusive changes in some patients with rheumatoid arthritis occur without evidence of clinical ischemia.

Primary Raynaud's disease

Arteriographic studies in patients with primary Raynaud's disease are difficult to perform because of vasospasm. This vasospasm must be avoided or released to ascertain the underlying state of the vasculature. Laws and co-workers (1963) found occlusive digital artery lesions in six of nine patients with Raynaud's phenomenon unassociated with connective tissue diseases. Porter and co-workers (1975) observed digital arterial disease in 14 of 16 patients with secondary Raynaud's phenomenon but no lesions in five patients with the primary disease; however, in a second report (1976), nine primary patients had diseased arteries although of less severity than the 32 patients with the secondary phenomenon. Jeune and Thivolet

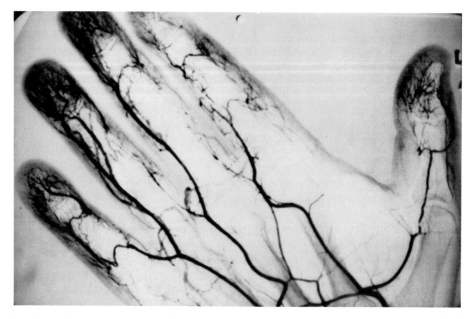

Fig. 3–1. Arteriogram of the finger blood vessels in a 29-year-old man with sclero-derma and severe Raynaud's phenomenon. The digital arteries of the second and fifth fingers are completely obstructed and the blood supply is by collateral vessels. The lateral digital arteries of the thumb, third, and fourth fingers are also severely diseased or obstructed.

(1978) observed normal arteriograms in all 11 patients who had Raynaud's phenomenon without underlying connective tissue disease.

SUMMARY

Only one histologic study has examined the digital arteries in two patients with mild primary Raynaud's disease and found no obvious abnormalities. In more severe cases, intimal hyperplasia, narrowing of the arterial lumen, and thrombi may occur. Angiographic studies also may be normal or demonstrate stenoses and occlusions of the digital arteries. With scleroderma and other secondary causes of Raynaud's phenomenon, pathology studies and angiography show digital artery stenoses and occlusions. With scleroderma the ulnar and radial arteries may be stenosed or occluded. Ultrastructural studies of the fingertip skin have demonstrated a variety of abnormalities of the capillaries, arteriovenous anastomoses, and nerves in primary and secondary Raynaud's phenomenon, but whether these changes are part of the disease process or secondary trophic effects due to the ischemia is as yet unknown.

REFERENCES

Bauer M, Hopfel-Kreiner I, Schlogel R: Funktionelle und morphologische vergleichende Untersuchungen der Durchklutung von Handen mit Dupuytrenscher Kontraktur und Raynaud-Syndrom. *Z Kardiol* 68:711, 1979.

Bollinger A, Jager K, Siegenthaler W: Microangiopathy of progressive systemic sclerosis. *Arch Intern Med* 146:1541, 1986.

Burch GE, Harb JM, Sun CS: Fine structure of digital vascular lesions in Raynaud's phenomenon and disease. *Angiology* 30:361, 1979.

Dabich L, Bookstein JJ, Zweifler A, Zarafonetis CJD: Digital arteries in patients with scleroderma. *Arch Intern Med* 130:708, 1972.

Jeune R, Thivolet J: Etude arteriographique de la main au cours de 52 phenomenes de Raynaud d'etiologie diverse. *Nouve Presse Med* 7:2619, 1978.

Laws JW, El Sallab RA, Scott JT: An arteriographic and histologic study of digital arteries. *Br J Radiol* 40:740, 1967.

Laws JW, Lillie JG, Scott JT: Arteriographic appearances in rheumatoid arthritis and other disorders. *Br J Radiol* 36:477, 1963.

Lewis T: The pathological changes in the arteries supplying the fingers in warm-handed people and in cases of so-called Raynaud's disease. *Clin Sci* 3:288, 1938.

Porter JM, Bardana EJ Jr, Bauer GM, Wesche DH, Andrasch RH, Rosch J: The clinical significance of Raynaud's phenomenon. *Surgery* 80:756, 1976.

Porter JM, Snider RL, Bardana EJ Jr, Rosch J, Eidemiller LR: The diagnosis and treatment of Raynaud's phenomenon. *Surgery* 77:11, 1975.

Rodnan GP, Myerowitz RL, Justh GO: Morphological changes in the digital arteries of patients with progressive systemic sclerosis (scleroderma) and Raynaud's phenomenon. *Medicine* 59:393, 1980.

Thompson RP, Harper FE, Maize JC, Ainsworth SK, LeRoy EC, Maricq HR: Nailfold biopsy in scleroderma and related disorders. *Arthritis Rheum* 27:97, 1984.

Vajda K, Kadar A, Kali A, Urai L: Ultrastructural investigations of finger pulp biopsies: a study of 31 patients with Raynaud's syndrome. *Ultrastruct Pathol* 3:175, 1982.

4

Pathophysiology

The pathophysiology of Raynaud's phenomenon has been difficult to study, as the vasospastic attacks are not easily induced in the laboratory, especially in patients with the primary disease. We have unsuccessfully tried to induce attacks using a combination of vasoconstrictor stimuli including total body cooling, local cooling, and intravenous norepinephrine infusions in patients with primary Raynaud's disease. Lewis (1929) immersed the hands of patients with the primary disease in 15°C water for 10 to 15 minutes; it produced cyanotic digits, but in colder water (0°–10°C) vasospastic phenomenon did not occur. Others have reported little difference between normal subjects and patients with primary Raynaud's disease during immersion in 0° to 2°C water (Thompson, 1959).

Induction of attacks of well demarcated color changes in the digits must be differentiated from the diffuse cyanosis easily produced in some patients with connective tissue disease or acrocyanosis, as different mechanisms are probably involved. It is likely that the well demarcated color changes are due to digital arterial spasm or closure, whereas diffuse changes are secondary to arteriolar vasoconstriction. This differentiation is important when analyzing investigative studies that claim to induce vasospastic attacks consistently in patients with the primary disease.

Raynaud's phenomenon has been attributed to overactivity of the sympathetic nervous system or abnormal sensitivity of the digital arteries to cold. These two theories have been the subject of many investigations since Raynaud's original description in 1888. The evidence for and against each proposal is presented herein (Table 4–1), and other possible pathogenetic mechanisms are discussed as well.

SYMPATHETIC NERVOUS SYSTEM

Raynaud (1888), describing the vasospastic disorder, considered that overactivity of the sympathetic nervous system was at fault; however, support for this theory has not been substantial. Interruption of the sympathetic nerves to the lower extremities often cures vasospastic attacks of the toes. Upper extremity sympathectomy, however, has not been successful, although it has not been performed on

Table 4–1. Pathophysiology Theories for Primary Raynaud's Disease

Sympathetic nervous system overactivity
    Sympathectomy may stop vasospastic attacks in toes
    Emotional stimuli may induce attacks
    Normal hand blood flow during heating
    Normal digital capillary flow with α-adrenoceptor blockade
    Increased catecholamines in wrist venous blood
    Exaggerated vasoconstrictor response to postural changes
Against sympathetic nervous system overactivity
    Local cooling of one hand does not increase reflex sympathetic vasoconstriction in the opposite hand
    Normal central thermoregulatory responses
    No increased sensitivity of digital blood flow to intravenous norepinephrine
    Normal plasma and urinary catecholamines in primary Raynaud's disease and scleroderma
    Normal cutaneous sympathetic nerve activity
    Digital vasodilatation during mental stress
Abnormal sensitivity of digital blood vessels to cold
    Local cooling produces ischemic attacks in single fingers
    Local cooling induces attacks in sympathetically denervated fingers
    Loss of digital systolic blood pressure with a local ischemic-cold stimulus
    Enhancement of reflex sympathetic vasoconstriction by local hand cooling
Generalized vasospasm
    Migraine headaches, variant angina, and Raynaud's phenomenon in some patients
    Pulmonary hypertension and Raynaud's phenomenon
Platelets
    No increase in plasma β-thromboglobulin or platelet aggregates
    No increase in prostaglandin I_2 or thromboxane A_2 metabolites
    Increased factor VIII/von Willebrand factor antigen or activity
Serotonin
    Serotonin inhibitors decrease intensity and duration of vasospastic attacks
    Increased plasma and intraplatelet serotonin in primary and secondary Raynaud's phenomenon
    Intraarterial serotonin produces a reddish hand
    Serotonin S_2 receptor inhibitor does not prevent cold-induced vasoconstriction
Abnormality of cold-induced vasodilatation
    Cold vasodilatation present but attenuated
Blood viscosity
    Contradictory studies regarding increased blood and plasma viscosity in primary Raynaud's disease
Systemic and finger arterial blood pressure
    Decreased systemic blood pressure in primary Raynaud's disease
    Decreased digital artery transmural pressure
Hereditary or familial factor
β-Adrenoceptors
Corticosteroids
Thermal entrainment

a group of patients with very early primary Raynaud's disease. In support of this theory is the fact that emotional stimuli produce vasospastic attacks in some patients.

Studies by Peacock (1957, 1959a) tended to substantiate the presence of excess sympathetic activity. An abnormally low average hand blood flow (plethysmography) of 2.9 ml·min^{-1} 100 ml^{-1} of tissue was found in a group of patients with primary Raynaud's disease in a 20°C room with the hand in 32°C water compared to a blood flow of 6.3 ml in normal subjects. After sympathetic inhibition by body warming with the hand in 42°C water, hand blood flow rose to normal levels (30.5 ml in patients versus 36 ml in normal subjects). Jamieson and co-workers (1971) have reported similar findings for hand flow. Olsen and co-workers (1987) reported that the vasoconstrictor response of digital blood flow (radioisotope disappearance rate) to venous stasis was normal in patients with primary Raynaud's disease or vibration-induced vasospastic disease, but both groups showed an exaggerated vasoconstrictor response to postural changes. These authors concluded that there was hyperreactivity of the central sympathetic nervous system to orthostatic stress but a normal axonal reflex. Since the vasoconstrictor response of fingers exposed to vibration was greater in women with primary Raynaud's disease than normal controls and could be abolished by proximal nerve blockade, Olsen and Petring (1988) came to the same conclusion. The normal vasodilatation in patients with primary Raynaud's disease rules against structural arterial disease and implicates the sympathetic nervous system control of blood vessel tone in the lower blood flow that occurs in a cool environment.

Fig. 4–1. Total and capillary fingertip blood flows are significantly smaller in patients with Raynaud's phenomenon (●) than in normal subjects (O) in a warm and cool room. There is a significant decrease in total blood flow with body cooling in both patients and normal subjects, but only capillary blood flow decreases in the patients. *Source:* Coffman and Cohen (1971).

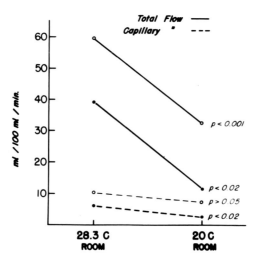

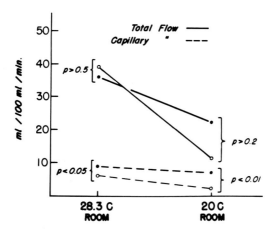

Fig. 4–2. Total fingertip blood flow is not significantly affected by reserpine treatment in a warm or a cool room. Capillary blood flow is significantly increased in both environments, and it decreases significantly with body cooling before but not during treatment. (O) before reserpine. (●) after reserpine. *Source:* Coffman and Cohen (1971).

We have found that finger blood flow (plethysmography) is significantly smaller in patients with primary and secondary Raynaud's phenomenon than in normal subjects in a warm (28.3°C) environment and in a 20°C room (Fig. 4–1) (Coffman and Cohen, 1971). The decreased fingertip flow has been confirmed by others (Cristol et al., 1979; Ohgi et al., 1985). However, in a study by Bollinger and Schlumpf (1976), the lower fingertip blood flow (plethysmography) of patients with primary Raynaud's disease did not reach statistical significance when compared to that of normal subjects in a 24°C room. We also found that capillary blood flow (radioisotope disappearance rate) in the finger was significantly less in both warm and cool environments in patients with primary and secondary Raynaud's phenomenon compared to that in normal subjects, but the flow could be normalized by α-adrenoceptor blockade with reserpine (Fig. 4–2) (Coffman and Cohen, 1971).

Against the hypothesis of overactivity of the sympathetic nervous system is the fact that Downey and Frewin (1973) failed to find increased reflex sympathetic vasoconstriction by locally cooling one hand while measuring blood flows in the opposite hand (plethysmography) in patients with Raynaud's phenomenon, probably of the primary type. Also, an increased sensitivity to cold was not present in the cooled hand of patients compared to normal subjects. Downey and co-workers (1971) reported a normal central thermoregulatory response in the hand (calorimetry) to increases or decreases in central body temperature in patients with primary disease but failure to vasodilate in the hand during central heating in patients with secondary Raynaud's phenomenon. Mendlowitz and Naftchi (1959) did find a heightened digital vasomotor tone (calorimetry), perhaps due to increased sympathetic neural discharge, but only in some patients with primary Raynaud's disease. They could not demonstrate increased sensitivity of digital blood flow to intravenous norepinephrine.

Peacock (1959b) measured increased catecholamine levels in wrist venous blood of patients with primary Raynaud's disease. The increase in catecholamines was postulated to originate in the sympathetic nerve endings of the extremities and was considered evidence for continuous sympathetic vasoconstrictor overactivity. Peacock also found an absence of monoamine oxidase in the digital artery of an amputated finger from one patient, indicating that a failure of metabolism of the catecholamines may be present. This finding would be more in favor of a local fault at the digital artery level. However, the enzyme catechol-o-methyltransferase also metabolizes catecholamines and was not measured. Using more refined techniques and carefully controlled studies, elevated plasma and urinary catecholamine levels have not been confirmed in primary Raynaud's disease (Kontos and Wasserman, 1969) or in Raynaud's phenomenon due to scleroderma (Sapira et al., 1972).

Naide and Sayen (1946) postulated that venospasm was important in the induction of vasospastic attacks, as veins were small and venous pressure could not be measured in the arm during room cooling. However, Landis (1929) dismissed venospasm as a factor. He demonstrated, by microinjection studies of capillary blood pressure in patients with primary Raynaud's disease, that the pressure rose little and slowly in response to venous congestion and fell rapidly with release of the congeston during body cooling.

Microelectrode recordings of skin sympathetic nerve activity do not demonstrate an abnormality in patients with primary Raynaud's disease (Fagius and Blumberg, 1985). These recordings were made from the median nerve supplying the hand in warm subjects during ice water immersion of the contralateral hand and other stimuli. Neither hypersensitivity of the vessels to strong sympathetic bursts nor an abnormal increase in sympathetic outflow was found. This study provides strong evidence against the theory of overactivity of the sympathetic nervous system in primary Raynaud's disease.

Because psychic stress has frequently been cited as a stimulus to vasospastic attacks, we studied fingertip blood flow (plethysmography) before and during a stressful mental task consisting of rapid serial arithmetic calculations in a 25°C room (Halperin et al., 1983). Significant elevations in heart rate and blood pressure indicated that stress was indeed induced in a group of patients with primary Raynaud's disease and in normal subjects. During mental stress in normal subjects, blood flow decreased (46.4 ± 6.2 to 22.4 ± 4.9 ml·min^{-1} 100 ml^{-1} tissue; $p < 0.01$) and vascular resistance increased (2.1 ± 0.4 to 7.6 ± 2.2 units, $p < 0.01$) (Fig. 4–3). Patients with primary Raynaud's disease unexpectedly had increased blood flow (15.4 ± 4.2 to 21.6 ± 5.7 ml; $p = 0.05$) and decreased vascular resistance (9.7 ± 2.3 to 7.1 ± 1.4 units; $p = 0.05$). Ten normal subjects studied in a cool room remained vasoconstricted during stress (blood flow 7.4 ± 2.9 to 5.1 ± 1.3 ml). The digital vasodilatation that occurred during mental stress in patients with primary Raynaud's disease was not altered by pretreatment with oral indomethacin, intraarterial propranolol or atropine, or digital nerve block. The results of this study argue against a role of the sympathetic nervous system in primary Raynaud's disease. However, the laboratory-controlled mental arithmetic task and unplanned emotional upset may represent dissimilar stressful stimuli.

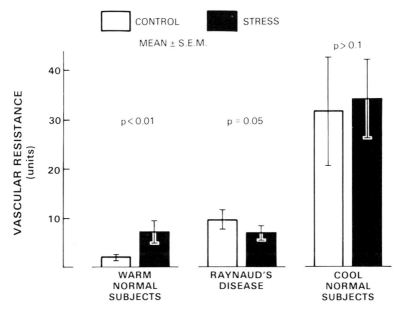

Fig. 4–3. Average fingertip vascular resistance before and during mental arithmetic stress in ten normal subjects and ten patients with primary Raynaud's disease. Vasoconstriction occurred in normal subjects, whereas vasodilatation was seen in the patients. Cool normal subjects showed no change. *Source:* Halperin et al., 1983. Reprinted by permission of Cardiovascular Research, British Medical Association House.

LOCAL FAULT

The "local fault" theory proposes that the blood vessels are abnormally sensitive to cold. Lewis (1929) studied a small group of patients with primary Raynaud's disease and demonstrated that local cooling produced ischemic attacks in single fingers and sympathetically denervated fingers. Furthermore, vasospasm during attacks in the fifth finger was not relieved by anesthetizing the ulnar nerve. Usually this procedure produced vasodilation of vessels by inhibiting vasoconstrictor tone. Lewis therefore concluded that local hypersensitivity to cold was present. Because attacks could be resolved by proximal (but not distal) warming of the finger, and a vasospastic attack could occur with proximal cooling of a finger with the tip kept warm, it was surmised that the digital artery, not the arterioles, were involved. In more severe cases, Lewis considered that intimal thickening and thrombosis of digital vessels contributed to the diminished blood flow. In this regard, his detailed observations have been criticized in that they were mostly made using patients with far advanced disease, and so structural changes may have been present in the digital vessels. Many of his patients had associated diseases and would not be classified as having the primary disease by current diagnostic techniques; however, his observations bear repeating on a more rigidly selected group of patients. Halpern and co-workers (1960) were also able to produce vasospastic attacks in patients with primary and secondary Raynaud's phenomenon despite acute sympathetic blocks of the extremities. Digital artery vasospasm during cold exposure is substantiated by the studies of Nielsen (1978). He showed that in patients with primary Raynaud's disease the digital systolic pressure can fall to zero when fingers are made ischemic and cooled to temperatures below 15°C, whereas normal subjects show a gradual reduction in systolic pressure.

Additional evidence in support of the local fault theory is that reflex sympathetic vasoconstriction is enhanced in patients with primary Raynaud's disease or scleroderma by locally cooling the hand but not in normal subjects (Jamieson et al., 1971). Hand blood flows were measured by plethysmography with one hand at 26°C and the other at 36°C while the body was heated to the point of sweating. The sympathetic stimulus was ice application to the neck for 30 seconds. Jamieson et al. considered that the most likely explanation of the greater decrease in flow of the cooled hand in patients was that cold temperatures sensitize the α-adrenoceptor-mediated vasoconstriction of vascular smooth muscle. A similar cold sensitivity of the α-adrenoceptors has now been shown to be present in canine saphenous veins (Janssens and Vanhoutte, 1978).

Keenan and Porter (1983) reported increased levels of α_2-adrenoceptors of platelets using a direct binding assay in patients with primary Raynaud's disease, in contrast to the number in control subjects and in patients with secondary Raynaud's phenomenon with digital artery obstruction. Binding capacity and affinity of α_2-adrenoceptors of platelets were later measured in patients with primary and secondary Raynaud's phenomenon and found to be increased only in patients with the primary disease (Edward et al., 1987). However, at least one-fourth of the patients had values that were less than the mean value of normal subjects. The α_2-adrenoceptor levels of platelets from normal subjects decreased after incubation with serum from patients with primary Raynaud's disease. The authors suggested the possibility of receptor modulation as a mechanism for increased cellular receptor synthesis. These studies are difficult to interpret, as varying levels of receptor number and activity were found in patients and normal subjects. Elevated α_2-adrenoceptor activity levels could mean that the reactivity of blood vessels to receptor agonists is increased and is a mechanism of vasospasm. α_2-Adrenoceptors have not yet been measured in tissues of Raynaud's phenomenon patients to demonstrate a correlation with the levels measured in platelet studies.

GENERALIZED VASOSPASM

A strong correlation of Raynaud's phenomenon and migraine headaches in patients with variant angina was reported by Miller and co-workers (1981). Fifteen of 62 patients with variant angina had Raynaud's phenomenon, whereas only 3 of 62 patients with other forms of coronary artery disease and 2 of 62 controls had vasospastic attacks. Migraine headaches occurred in 16 of the 62 variant angina patients but in only 4 and 6 of the two control groups, respectively. These differences were all statistically significant. Seven patients had all three entities; none of the controls had them; and 24 patients with variant angina had one of the two other conditions. The coincidence of the three syndromes suggests that a systemic factor causes vasospasm in the digital, cerebral, and coronary vasculature. It could be a blood-borne or neurologic factor or a generalized functional abnormality of vascular smooth muscle (Coffman and Cohen, 1981). Another coincidence that possibly includes vasospasm in more than one system is the rare condition of pulmonary hypertension with Raynaud's phenomenon but no underlying systemic disease (see Chap. 6). Vasospasm has not been demonstrated in the pulmonary vessels of patients with this disease, but pathological abnormalities to account for the pulmonary hypertension are often absent.

Raynaud's phenomenon is due to a spasm of digital arteries; a decrease in cerebral regional blood flow evidently due to vasoconstriction precedes migraine headaches; and coronary artery vasospasm has been shown angiographically to occur in patients with variant angina. With scleroderma, a disease commonly manifesting Raynaud's phenomenon, a generalized vascular abnormality predisposing to vasospasm may occur, as patients who die of myocardial infarction may have normal coronary arteries, and left ventricular dysfunction (Ellis et al., 1986) and decreased renal cortical blood flow (Cannon et al., 1974) have been described with body cooling or a cold pressor stimulus. It is known that patients with migraine headaches and primary Raynaud's disease have some abnormal peripheral vascular reactions to physiological stimuli. Patients with migraine headaches do not have normal vasodilatation in their hands when their body is heated (Appenzeller et al., 1963); patients with primary Raynaud's disease have vasodilatation instead of vasoconstriction in their fingers during mental stress (Halperin et al., 1983). Finally, emotional stress is an established precipitant of both Raynaud's phenomenon and migraine headaches.

One problem with the theory of a generalized vascular abnormality causing vasospasm is the difference in the neurogenic control of the three circulations. Sympathetic control of the circulation is greatest in the digital blood vessels, less in the coronary arteries, and negligible in the cerebral arteries. However, the vessels in the three circulations could respond with vasospasm because of their type of receptor predominance or because of unknown local factors.

β-ADRENOCEPTORS

Giovanni and co-workers (1984) infused isoprenaline 0.2 mg i.v. into 15 patients with primary Raynaud's disease and normal controls while performing digital photoelectric plethysmography. There was a highly significant decrease in pulse volume in the patients compared to controls. These investigators hypothesized that the vasoconstriction may be due to hypersensitivity of presynaptic β-adrenoceptors, increasing the liberation of norepinephrine from nerve terminals. These studies must be repeated with more exact methods of measuring blood flow and then the mechanism determined if an abnormality is found.

CORTICOSTEROIDS

Surwit and co-workers (1983) found higher levels of cortisol in brachial venous blood during environmental cold exposure of patients with Raynaud's phenomenon who had negative tests for antinuclear antibodies (ANA) than in ANA-positive patients and normal controls. The ANA-negative patients also had lower plasma norepinephrine levels. Surwit et al. hypothesized that the high levels of cortisol may be responsible for the vasospastic attacks, as glucocorticoids have been shown to increase vasomotor reactivity to norepinephrine. However, this theory would conflict with the failure to find an increased pressor response to intravenous norepinephrine (Coffman, unpublished observations; Mendlowitz and Naftchi, 1959) or decreased catecholamine levels in patients by other investigators (Kontos and Wasserman, 1969).

THERMAL ENTRAINMENT

Lafferty and co-workers (1983a) have shown that thermal entrainment, i.e., stimulation of the hypothalamus through the sympathetic stimulus of local temperature changes of a hand, is abnormal in patients with Raynaud's phenomenon (etiologies unknown). When one hand is alternately warmed and cooled, the blood vessels in the other hand vasodilate and vasoconstrict rapidly in normal subjects, but in patients with Raynaud's phenomenon the rapid vasodilatation is delayed or absent. In normal subjects, H_1 and H_2 histaminergic receptor blocking agents produce attenuation of the vasodilatation similar to that seen in patients with Raynaud's phenomenon (Lafferty et al., 1983b). These investigators hypothesized that there is a local fault in the histaminergic vasodilating system in patients with Raynaud's phenomenon. However, a neurogenic vasodilating mechanism has not been shown in human fingers, and a role for histamine in the physiological control of finger blood flow has not been determined.

PLATELETS

Platelets obtained from patients with Raynaud's phenomenon of various etiologies have been reported to be significantly more responsive to epinephrine than platelets from normal subjects; the platelets also produce more thromboxane A_2 and are resistant to prostaglandin inhibitors of platelet aggregation (Hutton et al., 1984). However, both normal subjects and patients had platelets more resistant to prostaglandin inhibitors when reactions were carried out at 27°C than when done at 37°C. Patients also had increased plasma levels of β-thromboglobulin, fibrinogen, and circulating platelet aggregates. Cooling of the forearms had the same effect on platelet function tests in normal subjects and patients. Other investigators have found increased plasma β-thromboglobulin levels and platelet aggregates in patients with scleroderma but not in those with primary Raynaud's disease or systemic lupus erythematosus (Dorsch and Meyerhoff, 1980; Kahaleh et al., 1982; Seibold and Harris, 1985).

β-Thromboglobulin levels in plasma are considered to represent the degree of activation or aggregation of platelets. Elevated levels are present in a number of conditions associated with microvascular disease or intravascular coagulation. Platelet factor 4, which is also a measure of the platelet release reaction, was not increased in a mixed group of patients with Raynaud's phenomenon in one study (Hutton et al., 1984) but was high in patients with scleroderma in another study (Seibold and Harris, 1985).

Prostaglandins E_1 and E_2 and thromboxane B_2 levels were reported at extremely high levels in the plasma of patients with Raynaud's phenomenon due to scleroderma (Horrobin et al., 1983). There was no overlap with the levels found in normal subjects. Two groups of investigators (Belch et al., 1985; Kinney and Demers, 1981) found levels of the metabolites of prostaglandin I_2 (prostacyclin) to be elevated and the red blood cell rigidity increased in patients with scleroderma but not in those with primary Raynaud's disease. The importance of these findings is yet to be elucidated. Treatment with indomethacin had no effect on the Raynaud's phenomenon (Kinney and Demers, 1981). This group found no elevation in plasma thromboxane B_2, whereas other investigators (Reilly et al., 1986) reported that the urinary metabolites of thromboxane A_2 and prostacyclin were elevated and increased further with cooling in patients with scleroderma. Factor VIII/ von Willebrand factor antigen and von Willebrand factor activity have been found to be increased in the blood of patients with primary Raynaud's disease and scleroderma (Kahaleh et al., 1981); it was postulated to reflect endothelial cell injury. Endothelial cell injury may presage the development of structural vascular disease, but its role in the pathogenesis of primary Raynaud's disease is unknown.

A role for platelets in the pathogenesis of Raynaud's phenomenon, especially the primary disease, has not been defined. Platelets could play a secondary role by aggravating vasospasm or occluding small vessels when microvascular disease is already present. If they played a major role, antiplatelet agents or drugs that block the effects of platelet vasoconstrictor products, e.g., thromboxane A_2 inhibitors or serotonin antagonists, should be more effective in the treatment of Raynaud's phenomenon than has been shown so far.

SEROTONIN

Serotonin has become increasingly implicated in the pathogenesis of vasospasm, especially in the coronary arteries. The serotonin could be derived from platelets or even serotonergic nerves. Halpern and co-workers (1960) reported that methysergide, a serotonin inhibitor, reduced the intensity and duration of the response of their patients with primary Raynaud's disease to immersion of the hands in cold water, although blanching still occurred. Moreover, intraarterial injection of serotonin (15 μg/min) and cooling of the hand produced an intensified vasoconstrictor effect. Serotonin injections produced a reddish hand that with prolonged infusions turned blue and whose digital temperature decreased; the effect was not inhibited by sympathetic nerve blockade. Whether any of the patients in this study had primary Raynaud's disease is questionable, as other investigators have been unable to consistently produce vasospastic attacks by immersing the hands in cold water (15°C).

Vascular smooth muscle strips from subcutaneous wrist vessels of three of four patients with scleroderma were reported to be hypersensitive to serotonin but not to catecholamines (Winkelmann, 1976). This increased sensitivity did not correlate with endothelial fibrosis. The demonstration that the subcutaneous injection of serotonin produces prolonged vasoconstriction in hands of patients with scleroderma compared to that in normal subjects would correlate with this report (Scherbel and Harrison, 1959).

Biondi and co-workers (1988) measured plasma free and intraplatelet serotonin in 30 patients with Raynaud's phenomenon of various etiologies. Plasma serotonin was elevated, compared to normal controls, in primary and secondary Raynaud's phenomenon and was highest in the patients with the secondary form. Platelet serotonin was also elevated, but equally in the primary and secondary type patients. This increased circulating serotonin could be due to continuous platelet activation. The reason for increased platelet serotonin is unknown, but it could be due to increased uptake with the high plasma levels. Whether the increased plasma serotonin levels are of pathogenetic importance or result from vascular disease in the small blood vessels remains to be determined.

There are several problems with implicating serotonin as having a primary role in the pathogenesis of Raynaud's phenomenon. Intraarterially administered vasoconstrictor doses of serotonin do not produce blanching of the fingers but, rather, an erythematous bluish discoloration (Coffman and Cohen, 1988; Halpern et al., 1960; Roddie et al., 1955). Administration of ketanserin, an S_2-serotonergic blocking agent, to patients with Raynaud's phenomenon in chronic studies has produced variable results (see Chap. 7). Also, acute administration of ketanserin did not prevent cold-induced vasoconstriciton, although it did relieve similar vasoconstriction already induced (Seibold and Terregino, 1986). Ketanserin is an α_1-adrenoceptor antagonist, which could explain some of its vasodilating action (Van Nueten et al., 1981). Before the role of serotonin in digital vasospasm can be clarified, more specific S_2-serotonergic blocking agents and agents that block the other serotonergic receptors must be studied in patients.

COLD-INDUCED VASODILATATION

Thompson (1959) studied cold-induced vasodilatation (see Chap. 1) in patients with primary and secondary Raynaud's phenomenon by measuring digital blood flow (calorimetry) during finger immersion in 0° to 2°C water. In mild cases the response was similar to that in normal subjects, but in the more severe cases the initial cold-induced vasodilatation was often delayed and reduced in amplitude. Marshall and co-workers (1953) also showed that cold-induced vasodilatation was present in patients with primary Raynaud's disease (see Fig. 1–8). Using calorimetry as an indication of blood flow, Magos and Okos (1963) studied cold-induced vasodilatation in normal subjects, patients with Raynaud's phenomenon never exposed to vibration, and patients with vibration-induced vasospastic disease by exposing fingers to 9.5°C water temperature. The vasodilatation that follows the initial vasoconstriciton was delayed and less marked in the patients. Magos and Okos considered that Raynaud's phenomenon may not be due to cold sensitivity but, rather, to a defect in the cold-induced vasodilatation.

Cold-induced vasodilatation has also been studied in patients with primary Raynaud's disease using 5°, 10°, and 15°C water immersion of one finger (Jobe et al., 1985). At 10° and 15°C, there were some differences in the patients; i.e., there were fewer vasodilatation cycles and a lesser rise in digital temperature compared to the normal subjects. The authors concluded that cold aggravates an abnormality already present at higher temperatures or adds a second abnormality.

Therefore cold vasodilatation occurs in patients with Raynaud's phenomenon, although it may be attenuated. The difference from normal subjects does not add to our understanding of the pathophysiology of the disease.

BLOOD VISCOSITY

The possibility has been raised that intravascular coagulation may be involved in the pathogenesis of primary Raynaud's disease. Because patients with cryoglobulinemia have increased blood, plasma, and serum viscosity and develop Raynaud's phenomenon, hyperviscosity as a factor in the primary disease appears to be a reasonable hypothesis. However, studies of blood or plasma viscosity in patients have been conflicting.

In 1965 Pringle and co-workers, using the free-flow bleeding method of Pirofsky in a 20°C room, reported that whole blood viscosity was twice as high in 22 patients with primary Raynaud's disease as in the control subjects. They also noted an increased fibrinogen level in 18 of the patients and found sludging of blood cells by capillary microscopy of the conjunctival vessels.

It is noteworthy that this method was not used to measure blood viscosity by other investigators who tried to confirm this study; instead, they used various kinds of viscometer. Goyle and Dormandy (1976) found that blood viscosity was significantly increased in patients with primary Raynaud's disease but only at a shear rate of 0.77 sec^{-1} at 27°C. There was no difference at a slightly higher shear rate or at 37°C. Jahnsen and associates (1977) reported an increase in blood viscosity in similar patients, only at a shear rate of 11.5 sec^{-1} at 27°C and not at higher (up to 230 sec^{-1}) or lower shear rates. Whole blood or plasma viscosity was found to be elevated at several shear rates by some investigators (Blunt et al., 1980; Walder, 1973).

McGrath and co-workers (1978) found normal blood viscosities at warm and cool temperatures despite reduced hand blood flows (plethysmography) in patients with primary Raynaud's disease. Other investigators have reported normal blood or plasma viscosity in patients with primary Raynaud's disease (Ayres et al., 1981; Sandhagen and Wegener, 1985; Sergio et al., 1983).

We have measured plasma and blood viscosities at moderate to high shear rates (75–1500 sec^{-1}) and low temperature (25°C) in 28 patients with primary Raynaud's disease and 29 patients with scleroderma (Creager and Coffman, 1977). Plasma viscosity was significantly increased at all shear rates in patients with scleroderma and in those with primary Raynaud's disease except at the highest shear rate. Blood viscosity was not elevated in either disease.

Studying scleroderma, McGrath and co-workers (1977) reported that 35 percent of patients had blood hyperviscosity at 35°C at a high shear rate (73 sec^{-1}) and 70 percent at a low shear rate (0.18 sec^{-1}). Other investigators have also found elevated plasma viscosity in patients with generalized connective tissue disorders (Ayres et al., 1981; Sergio et al., 1983; Tietjen and co-workers, 1975).

One of the most likely constituents of blood that would increase its viscosity is fibrinogen. However, high and normal fibrinogen levels have been reported in groups of patients with primary or secondary Raynaud's phenomenon (Creager and Coffman, 1977; Goyle and Dormandy, 1976; Jahnsen et al., 1977; Jamieson et al., 1971; Pringle et al., 1965; Tietjen et al., 1975). Jahnsen and colleagues (1977) treated five patients with primary disease with venesection to lower the hematocrit and the whole blood and plasma viscosity, but they detected no change in finger systolic blood pressure or its reaction to cold. Treatment with stanozolol decreased fibrinogen and increased the hematocrit; it caused no change in whole blood viscosity even though hand blood flow showed an increase in ten patients with primary or secondary Raynaud's phenomenon (Ayres et al., 1981).

Blood viscosity is probably not of primary pathogenetic importance in patients with primary Raynaud's disease or scleroderma. Unless cryoprecipitable proteins are present, a high blood viscosity should not be associated with cold-induced vasospastic attacks because the temperature coefficient for blood viscosity is small (Jamieson et al., 1971). However, the changes in plasma viscosity could be a contributing factor, especially in the microcirculation where the viscosity of plasma predominates over that of red blood cells. It is possible that patients with a low blood flow in the digits on exposure to cold or due to morphological abnormalities in the digital arteries could develop more severe ischemia if the blood or plasma viscosity were abnormal.

SYSTEMIC AND FINGER ARTERIAL PRESSURE

Thulesius (1976) reported that patients with primary Raynaud's disease had a lower brachial artery blood pressure than normal subjects. Patients with secondary Raynaud's phenomenon had blood pressures similar to those of the control subjects. Cohen and Coffman (1989) compared segmental finger and arm arterial blood pressures and finger blood flow in ten normal subjects and nine patients with primary Raynaud's disease. *Fingertip perfusion pressure* (COP; see Chap. 1), defined as the blood pressure that maintains flow against external compression, and blood flow were measured by a plethysmographic method. During reflex sympathetic vasoconstriction induced by body cooling and with the hand kept warm, mean brachial blood pressure, brachial and finger systolic pressures, and fingertip perfusion pressure in patients were significantly lower than in normal subjects (Fig. 4–4). Dig-

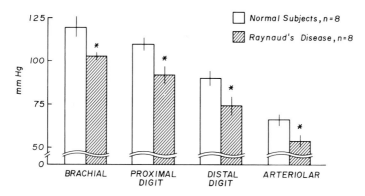

Fig. 4–4. Segmental systolic blood pressure measurements in normal subjects and patients with primary Raynaud's disease during reflex sympathetic vasoconstriction induced by body cooling. Brachial, proximal and distal digital, and arteriolar (critical opening) pressures were significantly lower in the patients than in the normal subjects (*$p < 0.05$). *Source:* Cohen RA, Coffman JD (1989).

ital nerve block caused no change in finger systolic pressure in either group, indicating that reflex sympathetic vasoconstriction was not the cause of the lower pressure in patients (Fig. 4–5). Following nerve blockade, perfusion pressure and blood flow increased equally in normal subjects and patients, suggesting similar degrees of sympathetic-nerve-mediated vasoconstriction of the small fingertip resistance vessels. These findings argue against the theory of an exaggerated reflex sympathetic nervous response to body cooling being at fault in Raynaud's disease.

The lower blood pressures in the arms and fingers of patients with Raynaud's disease may partially explain their predisposition to develop vasospasm, as transmural arterial distending forces are decreased and less external pressure is required to stop blood flow. However, it cannot be the entire pathophysiological problem, as not all patients have low pressures and not all subjects with low pressures develop vasospasm. In some patients however, the low pressures may contribute to the basic abnormality.

HEREDITARY OR FAMILIAL FACTOR

Raynaud's phenomenon may occur in several members of a family, raising the possibility of a hereditary or familial factor. This association has not been well documented in the literature but is mentioned by Goetz (1956) and Spittell (1972). We have seen occasional familial occurrences of vasospastic attacks in patients and their families involving mothers, fathers, or siblings. However, some of the patients involved in these familial occurrences had Raynaud's phenomenon due to different etiologies. Goetz (1956) also mentioned Raynaud's phenomenon secondary to different etiologies in the same family. It is doubtful that there is a hereditary factor

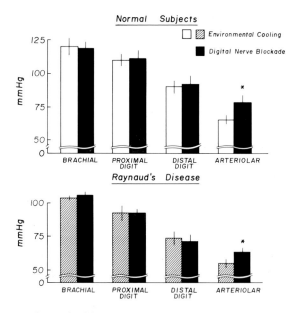

Fig. 4–5. Segmental systolic blood pressure measurements before and during digital nerve block in normal subjects and patients with primary Raynaud's disease. Reflex sympathetic vasoconstriction was induced by body cooling in these studies. The brachial, proximal, and distal digital systolic blood pressures were unchanged, whereas the critical opening pressure (arteriolar) was increased by the nerve block in both normal subjects and patients (*$p < 0.05$). *Source:* Cohen RA, Coffman JD (1989).

in primary Raynaud's disease, but there may be a genetic factor in some of the connective tissue diseases.

SUMMARY

Many factors have been implicated in the pathophysiology of vasospastic attacks of the digits (Fig. 4–6). Most of the secondary causes of Raynaud's phenomenon are associated with decreased blood flow or blood pressure in the digits. Digital artery stenoses or obstructions are usually seen with the connective tissue diseases, traumatic vasospastic disease, and some of the drug-induced syndromes and would cause low blood pressure in the distal vessels. Decreased digital blood flow would result from sludging of blood when hyperviscosity is present. With some of the connective tissue diseases and perhaps hypothyroidism, there may be narrowing of the vessel lumen by structural thickening or edema. In the obstructive arterial diseases, large-vessel obstruction causes low blood pressure in the distal digital vessels. The carpal tunnel syndrome and thoracic outlet syndromes, by constant sympathetic nerve irritation, and some of the drug etiologies may cause persistent digital artery vasoconstriction. It can then be envisioned that a low digital artery pressure, thickened vessel walls, increased blood viscosity, and persistent vasoconstriction along with the resulting release of vasoconstrictive products from the breakdown of platelets could, alone or in concert, lead to closure of small arteries during a normal sympathetic stimulus with or without an increase in extravascular pressure.

However, with the primary disease, structural abnormalities have not been demonstrated in the digital vessels. The strongest evidence indicates a local sensitivity of the digital arteries to cold, but the cause is unknown. Promising studies indicate that the abnormality may be in the α-adrenoceptors. It is possible that this dysfunction lies in the arteriovenous anastomoses that apparently control the finger blood flow response to body cooling via α_2-adrenoceptors (see Chap. 1). Raynaud's phenomenon occurs only in the body parts that contain arteriovenous anastomoses.

Many people have a rare vasospastic attack, usually in only one finger. These isolated events generally occur during cold exposure of both the body and the digits. It is probable that a combination of factors may induce digital artery closure in any individual in certain situations, including vasoconstriction due to local cold and reflex sympathetic activity, external pressure on the digit, low systemic blood pressure, and perhaps release of vasoactive compounds from platelets. However,

Fig. 4–6. Factors that affect the intravascular pressure, extravascular pressure, and vascular wall tone. Digital vasospasm may occur with a change in any of the entities, but it probably involves a combination of factors. *Source:* Courtesy of R.A. Cohen.

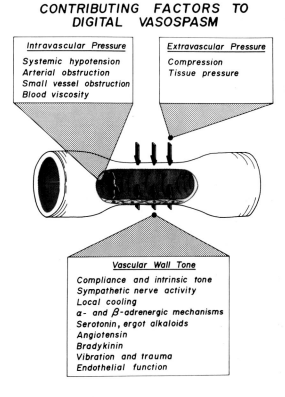

CONTRIBUTING FACTORS TO
DIGITAL VASOSPASM

Intravascular Pressure
Systemic hypotension
Arterial obstruction
Small vessel obstruction
Blood viscosity

Extravascular Pressure
Compression
Tissue pressure

Vascular Wall Tone
Compliance and intrinsic tone
Sympathetic nerve activity
Local cooling
a- and β-adrenergic mechanisms
Serotonin, ergot alkaloids
Angiotensin
Bradykinin
Vibration and trauma
Endothelial function

this theory does not explain the frequent daily attacks that occur in many patients with the primary disease. Thus there is still an important abnormality to be discovered.

REFERENCES

Appenzeller O, Davidson K, Marshall J: Reflex vasomotor abnormalities in the hands of migrainous subjects. *J Neurol Neurosurg Psychiatry* 26:477, 1963.

Ayres ML, Jarrett PEM, Browse NL: Blood viscosity, Raynaud's phenomenon and the effect of fibrinolytic enhancement. *Br J Surg* 68:51, 1981.

Belch JJF, McLaren M, Anderson J, Lowe GDO,Sturrock RD, Capell HA, Forbes CD: Increased prostacyclin metabolites and decreased red cell deformability in patients with systemic sclerosis and Raynaud's syndrome. *Prostaglandins Leukotrienes Med* 17:1, 1985.

Biondi ML, Marasini B, Bianchi E, Agostoni A: Plasma free and intraplatelet serotonin in patients with Raynaud's phenomenon. *Int J Cardiol* 19:335, 1988.

Blunt RJ, George AJ, Hurlow RA, Strachan CJL, Stuart J: Hyperviscosity and thrombotic changes in idiopathic and secondary Raynaud's phenomenon. *Br J Hematol* 45:651, 1980.

Bollinger A, Schlumpf M: Finger blood flow in healthy subjects of different age and sex and in patients with primary Raynaud's disease. *Acta Chir Scand* [Suppl] 465:42, 1976.

Cannon PJ, Hassar M, Case DP, Casarella WJ, Sommers SC, Leroy EC: The relationship of hypertension and renal failure in scleroderma (progressive systemic sclerosis) to structural and functional abnormalities of the renal cortical circulation. *Medicine* 53:1, 1974.

Coffman JD, Cohen AS: Total and capillary blood flow in Raynaud's phenomenon. *N Engl J Med* 285:259, 1971.

Coffman JD, Cohen RA: Vasospasm—ubiquitous? *N Engl J Med* 304:780, 1981.

Coffman JD, Cohen RA: Serotonergic vasoconstriction in human fingers during reflex sympathetic response to cooling. *Am J Physiol* 254:H889, 1988.

Cohen RA, Coffman JD: Reduced fingertip arterial pressure in Raynaud's disease. *J Vasc Med Biol* 1:21, 1989.

Creager MA, Coffman JD: Plasma and blood viscosity in Raynaud's phenomenon. *Clin Res* 25:214A, 1977.

Cristol R, Graisely B, Cloarec M, Debray J: Syndrome de Raynaud: etude du debit pulpaire digital par plethysmographie avec occlusion veineuse. *Nouv Presse Med* 8:105, 1979.

Dorsch C, Meyerhoff J: Elevated plasma β-thromboglobulin levels in systemic lupus erythematosus. *Thromb Res* 20:617, 1980.

Downey JA, Frewin DB: The effect of cold on blood flow in the hands of patients with Raynaud's phenomenon. *Clin Sci* 44:279, 1973.

Downey JA, LeRoy EC, Miller JM: Thermoregulation and Raynaud's phenomenon. *Clin Sci* 40:211, 1971.

Edward JM, Phinney ES, Taylor LM Jr., Keenan EJ, Porter JM: α_2-Adrenergic receptor levels in obstructive and spastic Raynaud's syndrome. *J Vasc Surg* 5:38, 1987.

Ellis WW, Baer AN, Robertson RM, Pincus T, Kronenberg MW: Left ventricular dysfunction induced by cold exposure in patients with systemic sclerosis. *Am J Med* 80:385, 1986.

Fagius J, Blumberg H: Sympathetic outflow to the hand in patients with Raynaud's phenomenon. *Cardiovasc Res* 19:249, 1985.

Giovanni B, Guiseppina CM, Susanna F, Roberto M: Altered regulator mechanisms of pre-synaptic adrenergic nerve: a new physiopathological hypothesis in Raynaud's disease. Microvasc Res 27:110, 1984.

Goetz RH: Raynaud's disease and Raynaud's phenomenon. In *Diagnosis and Treatment of Vascular Disorders*. Samuels SS (ed). Baltimore: Williams & Wilkins, 1956, p. 349.

Goyle KB, Dormandy JA: Abnormal blood viscosity in Raynaud's phenomenon. *Lancet* 1:1317, 1976.

Halperin JL, Cohen RA, Coffman JD: Digital vasodilatation during mental stress in patients with Raynaud's disease. *Cardiovasc Res* 17:671, 1983.

Halpern A, Kuhn P, Shaftel HE, Samuels SS, Schaftel N, Selman D, Birch HG: Raynaud's disease, Raynaud's phenomenon, and serotonin. *Angiology* 11:151, 1960.

Horrobin DF, Jenkins K, Manku MS: Raynaud's phenomenon, histamine, and prostaglandins. *Lancet* 2:747, 1983.

Hutton RA, Mikhailidis DP, Bernstein RM, Jeremy JY, Hughes GRV, Dandona P: Assessment of platelet function in patients with Raynaud's syndrome. *J Clin Pathol* 37:182, 1984.

Jahnsen T, Nielsen SL, Skovborg F: Blood viscosity and local response to cold in primary Raynaud's phenomenon. *Lancet* 2:1001, 1977.

Jamieson GG, Ludbrook J, Wilson A: Cold hypersensitivity in Raynaud's phenomenon. *Circulation* 44:254, 1971.

Janssens WJ, Vanhoutte PM: Instantaneous changes in alpha-adrenoceptor affinity caused by moderate cooling in canine cutaneous veins. *Am J Physiol* 234:330, 1978.

Jobe JB, Goldman RF, Beetham WP Jr: Comparison of the hunting reaction in normals and individuals with Raynaud's disease. *Aviat Space Environ Med* 56:568, 1985.

Kahaleh MB, Osborn I, LeRoy EC: Increased factor VIII/von Willebrand factor antigen and von Willebrand factor activity in scleroderma and in Raynaud's phenomenon. *Ann Intern Med* 94:482, 1981.

Kahaleh MB, Osborn I, LeRoy EC: Elevated levels of circulating platelet aggregates and beta-thromboglobulin in scleroderma. *Ann Intern Med* 96:610, 1982.

Keenan EJ, Porter JM: α_2-Adrenergic receptors in platelets from patients with Raynaud's syndrome. *Surgery* 94:204, 1983.

Kinney EL, Demers LM: Plasma 6-keto-PGF$_{1\alpha}$ concentration in Raynaud's phenomenon. *Prostaglandins Med* 7:389, 1981.

Kontos HA, Wasserman AJ: Effect of reserpine in Raynaud's phenomenon. *Circulation* 39:259, 1969.

Lafferty K, DeTrafford JC, Roberts VC, Cotton LT: Raynaud's phenomenon and thermal entrainment: an objective test. *Br Med J* 286:90, 1983a.

Lafferty K, DeTrafford JC, Roberts VC, Cotton LT: Raynaud's phenomenon: prostacyclin or histamine deficit? *Lancet* 1:536, 1983b.

Landis EM Jr: Micro-injection studies of capillary blood pressure in Raynaud's disease. *Heart* 15:247, 1929.

Lewis T: Experiments relating to the peripheral mechanism involved in spasmodic arrest of the circulation in the fingers, a variety of Raynaud's disease. *Heart* 15:7, 1929.

Magos L, Okos G: Cold dilatation and Raynaud's phenomenon. *Arch Environ Health* 7:402,1963.

Marshall RJ, Shepherd JT, Thompson ID: Vascular responses in patients with high serum titres of cold agglutinins. *Clin Sci* 12:255, 1953.

McGrath MA, Peck R, Penny R: Blood hyperviscosity with reduced skin blood flow in scleroderma. *Ann Rheum Dis* 36:569, 1977.

McGrath MA, Peck R, Penny R: Raynaud's disease: reduced hand blood flows with normal blood viscosity. *Aust NZ J Med* 8:126, 1978.

Mendlowitz M, Naftchi N: The digital circulation in Raynaud's disease. *Am J Cardiol* 4:580, 1959.

Miller D, Waters DD, Warnica W, Szlachcic J, Kreeft J, Theroux P: Is variant angina the coronary manifestation of a generalized vasospastic disorder? *N Engl J Med* 304:763, 1981.

Naide M, Sayen A: Venospasm. Arch Intern Med 77:16, 1946.

Nielsen SL: Raynaud phenomenon and finger systolic pressure during cooling. *Scand J Clin Lab Invest* 38:765, 1978.

Ohgi S, Moore DJ, Miles RD, Lambeth A, McAllister L, Sumner DS: The effect of cold on circulation in normal and cold sensitive fingers. *Bruit* 9:9, 1985.

Olsen N, Petring OU, Rossing N: Exaggerated postural vasoconstrictor reflex in Raynaud's phenomenon. *Br Med J* 294:1186, 1987.

Olsen N, Petring OU: Vibration elicited vasoconstrictor reflex in Raynaud's phenomena. *Br J Indust Med* 45:415, 1988.

Peacock JH: Vasodilatation in the human hand: observations on primary Raynaud's disease and acrocyanosis of the upper extremities. *Clin Sci* 17:575, 1957.

Peacock JH: A comparative study of the digital cutaneous temperatures and hand blood flows in the normal hand, primary Raynaud's disease, and primary acrocyanosis. *Clin Sci* 18:25, 1959a.

Peacock JH: Peripheral venous blood concentration of epinephrine and norepinephrine in primary Raynaud's disease. *Circ Res* 7:821, 1959b.

Pringle R, Walder DM, Weaver JPA: Blood viscosity and Raynaud's disease. *Lancet* 1:1086, 1965.

Raynaud M: *On Local Asphyxia and Symmetrical Gangrene of the Extremities.* Translated by T. Barlow. London: The Syndenham Society, 1888, p. 99.

Reilly IAG, Roy L, Fitzgerald GA: Biosynthesis of thromboxane in patients with systemic sclerosis and Raynaud's phenomenon. *Br Med J* 292:1037, 1986.

Roddie LC, Shepherd JT, Whelan RF: The action of 5-hydroxytryptamine on the blood vessels of the human hand and forearm. *Br J Pharmacol Chemother* 10:445, 1955.

Sandhagen B, Wegener T: Blood viscosity and finger systolic pressure in primary and traumatic vasospastic disease. *Ups J Med Sci* 90:55, 1985.

Sapira JD, Rodnan GP, Scheib ET, Klaniecki T, Rizk M: Studies of endogenous catecholamines in patients with Raynaud's phenomenon secondary to progressive systemic sclerosis (scleroderma). *Am J Med* 52:330, 1972.

Scherbel AL, Harrison JW: Response to serotonin and its antagonists in patients with rheumatoid arthritis and related diseases. *Angiology* 10:29, 1959.

Seibold JR, Harris JN: Plasma β-thromboglobulin in the differential diagnosis of Raynaud's phenomenon. *J Rheumatol* 12:99, 1985.

Seibold JR, Terregino CA: Selective antagonism of S_2-serotonergic receptors relieves but does not prevent cold-induced vasoconstriction in primary Raynaud's phenomenon. *J Rheumatol* 13:337, 1986.

Sergio G, Artale F, Francisci A, Giunti P, Perego MA: Emoreologia e sindromi acrali neurovascolari. *Ric Clin Lab* 13(suppl 3):481, 1983.

Spittell JA Jr: Raynaud's phenomenon and allied vasospastic conditions. In *Peripheral Vascular Diseases.* 4th Ed. Fairbairn JF II, Juergens JL, Spittell JA Jr (eds). Philadelphia: Saunders, 1972, p. 387.

Surwit RS, Allen LM, Gilgor RS, Schanberg S, Kuhn C, Duvic M: Neuroendocrine response to cold in Raynaud's syndrome. *Life Sci* 32:995, 1983.

Thompson ID: Vasospasm and cold. *Ir J Med Sci* 6:267, 1959.

Thulesius O: Methods for evaluation of peripheral vascular function in the upper extremities. *Acta Chir Scand* [Suppl] 465:53, 1976.

Tietjen GW, Chien S, LeRoy EC, Gavras I, Gavras H, Gump FE: Blood viscosity, plasma proteins, and Raynaud's syndrome. *Arch Surg* 110:1343, 1975.

Van Nueten JM, Janssen PAJ, Van Beek J, Xhonneaux R, Verbeuren TJ, Vanhoutte PM: Vascular effects of ketanserin (R 41 468), a novel antagonist of 5-HT$_2$ serotonergic receptors. *J Pharmacol Exp Ther* 218:217, 1981.

Walder DN: Blood viscosity and Raynaud's disease. *J R Coll Surg Edinb* 17:277, 1973.

Winkelmann RK, Goldyne ME, Linscheid RL: Hypersensitivity of scleroderma cutaneous vascular smooth muscle to 5-hydroxytryptamine. *Br J Dermatol* 95:51, 1976.

5

Diagnosis of Primary Raynaud's Disease

The diagnosis of vasospastic digital attacks is not difficult if the patient presents to the physician during an episode or clearly describes the dramatic clinical manifestations of episodic, well-demarcated digital color changes. The differential diagnosis of primary from secondary Raynaud's phenomenon, however, can be difficult. The history and physical exam can be helpful but interpretation of available tests is very important in the diagnosis of primary Raynaud's disease. Treatment and prognostic predictions for the patient depend on the physician's ability to arrive at the most likely diagnosis.

HISTORY AND PHYSICAL EXAMINATION

The diagnosis of Raynaud's phenomenon is usually easily made from a careful history. Vasospastic attacks are difficult to produce in the office or laboratory setting despite exposure to body cooling, digital cooling, intraarterial or intravenous norepinephrine, tobacco smoking, or mental stress (Coffman, personal observations). It is especially true of patients with the primary disease. Therefore the description of *episodic* attacks of *well demarcated* color changes of the digits on exposure to cold must often suffice for the diagnosis (see Fig. 2–1). The classic triad of white followed by first blue and then red digital color changes is dramatic but not always present; many patients experience only one or two of the ischemic color phases. The physical examination is normal in patients with the primary disease, although the hands or feet may be cool and demonstrate increased perspiration between attacks. Blood and urine studies are also normal in these patients.

Because vasospastic attacks may precede diagnostic criteria of connective tissue diseases, especially scleroderma, by several years, clinicians and investigators have relied on the criteria proposed by Allen and Brown (1932) for diagnosis of the primary disease.

1. Vasospastic attacks precipitated by exposure to cold or emotional stimuli
2. Bilateral involvement of the extremities
3. Absence of gangrene or, if present, limited to the skin of the fingertips

4. No evidence of an underlying disease that could be responsible for vasospastic attacks
5. History of symptoms for at least 2 years

These criteria are helpful, but some of the patients included here develop other
diseases, usually scleroderma, in the future. Fewer patients with connective tissue
diseases are missed if criterion 4 includes the absence of antinuclear antibodies and
a normal erythrocyte sedimentation rate (ESR), finger systolic blood pressures during local cold exposure, nailfold capillaroscopy, and esophageal motility studies.
However, this work-up is expensive and probably should be reserved for (1)
patients presenting with severe vasospastic attacks, ulcers, or gangrene; (2) men;
and (3) women who first develop the syndrome after age 40 (Coffman, 1985).
Although a large proportion of patients with Raynaud's phenomenon are reported
to have abnormal blood studies or other evidence of a secondary disease, these
studies emanate from university centers where the more severe cases are referred.
In the community the primary disease accounts for most cases, as evidenced by the
small incidence of connective tissue disease compared to the high frequency of
Raynaud's phenomenon in the general population. If a thorough history uncovers
no symptoms of secondary diseases or exposure to agents known to induce Raynaud's phenomenon, the physical examination is normal, and a complete blood
count, ESR, urinalysis, and chest film are normal in a woman 15 to 40 years of age,
the patient can be reassured she has a benign disease.

LABORATORY EXAMINATION

Finger Systolic Blood Pressure

Measurement of digital systolic blood pressures has been advocated to aid in the
diagnosis of Raynaud's phenomenon or digital artery obstructions. The measurements must be performed carefully (Kahlenbuhl et al., 1977). A thin-walled 2.4-cm
digital cuff gives the most exact measurements and is applied to the proximal part
of the digit (Fig. 5–1). The cuff is inflated above systolic blood pressure, which is
denoted by the absence of pulsations in the detection device used on the distal
finger to measure volume changes. Strain gauges, plethysmographs (volume, photoelectric), and spectroscopy have been used as detectors. The cuff is deflated at
approximately 2 mm/sec, and the first increase in finger volume indicates the systolic pressure. Digital pressure measurements should not be made during inflation
of the cuff at the cessation of pulsations, as a falsely high reading may be obtained.
The volume increase may be difficult to detect in vasoconstricted fingers, and careful positioning of the arm and hand above heart level, emptying of digital veins by
compression, and warming of the fingertip before the measurement may help. Finger systolic blood pressure is lower than arm systolic pressure by about 10 mm Hg
when the fingers are warm and dilated but rises to or toward arm pressure during
digital vasoconstriction. Downs and co-workers (1975) found that a difference of
more than 15 mm Hg between fingers, an absolute finger systolic blood pressure of
less than 70 mm Hg, or a wrist to digit gradient of more than 30 mm Hg in subjects

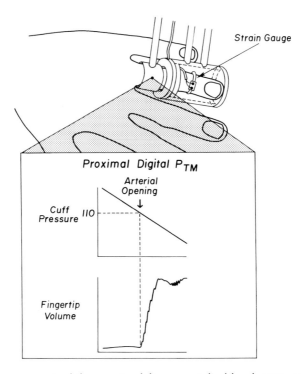

Fig. 5–1. Measurement of the proximal finger systolic blood pressure using a strain gauge to detect the increase in fingertip volume (P_{TM}) as the proximal cuff is slowly deflated from suprasystolic pressure. Fingertip pulsations and the volume increase are not detected until the cuff pressure deflates to 110 mm Hg, the point of digital artery opening. *Source:* Cohen RA, Coffman JD; unpublished observations.

with a warm hand (34°C) and body indicated organic obstruction of digital arteries as proved by arteriography. Similarly, Hirai (1978) found a correlation of low finger systolic blood pressure with obstructions of both digital arteries using arteriography. However, only 173 of 203 fingers with this radiological picture had a low finger systolic blood pressure, and fingers with one obstructed digital artery often had a normal finger systolic pressure.

Finger Systolic Blood Pressure and Cold Exposure

The effect of local cooling on finger systolic blood pressure has been used as a diagnostic test for Raynaud's phenomenon (Nielsen, 1978a). The digit is usually cooled by circulating water through a finger cuff around the proximal finger at 20°, 15°, 10°, and 5°C for 5-minute intervals. During the cooling the finger is made ischemic by inflating the digital blood pressure cuff to suprasystolic pressure, thereby aiding the finger to approximate the external temperature. Compared to normal subjects, patients with primary Raynaud's disease have a signfiicantly greater reduction in finger systolic blood pressure with cooling, and many patients show a loss of finger systolic pressure or digital arterial closure. Corbin and co-workers (1985) did not find this test of value for diagnosis because of low sensitivity, but they used a 2-minute cooling period. The diagnostic arterial closure is demonstrated in a greater proportion of patients if the body is also cooled with a cooling blanket or by exposure to an 18°C room (Hoare et al., 1982; Nielsen, 1978a). Carter and co-workers (1988) also found that body cooling in addition to local digital cooling was more likely to produce a large decrease or loss of finger systolic blood pressure in patients with Raynaud's phenomenon. In a study of 162 patients with Raynaud's phenomenon of various etiologies, 80 percent showed a positive test. Patients with secondary disease were more likely to have the abnormal finger systolic blood pressure response than those with primary disease. This finding was contrary to those in a study by Nielsen and colleagues (1978b), who reported that patients with Raynaud's phenomenon and proximal arterial obstruction of large arteries were less sensitive to local cooling than patients who had the primary disease without obstructions. However, the two groups of investigators were probably studying different patient populations. The day-to-day variation in finger systolic blood pressure is large, so that finger systolic pressure measurement may not be appropriate for longitudinal studies (Malamet et al., 1984). Also, as indicated previously, the point of increase in finger volume may be difficult to detect in cooled fingers. Finger systolic blood pressure and cold exposure does not differentiate the primary disease from secondary Raynaud's phenomenon.

Nailfold Capillary Microscopy

Nailfold capillary microscopy has been used for diagnosing Raynaud's phenomenon due to secondary causes. After the skin of the nailfold is cleansed with alcohol, a film of immersion oil is applied. The superficial blood vessels can then be visualized with a magnifying glass, ophthalmoscope, or a compound microscope with a cool light source. With the latter, a wide field and a magnification of ×10 or ×20 is usually recommended. Normally, the superficial capillaries are seen as regularly spaced, hairpin loops aligned along the axis of the digit; the subpapillary venous plexus can be seen in fewer than 10 percent of subjects (Fig. 5–2). One note of caution is that edema may blur the capillary pattern. Abnormalities consisting in enlarged and tortuous capillary loops, a sparsity of capillaries, and avascular areas may be seen in patients with connective tissue diseases. Hemorrhages may be present but also occur occasionally in normal individuals. The most diagnostic picture is seen in patients with scleroderma, mixed connective tissue disease, and dermatomyositis; it consists in enlarged, deformed capillary loops surrounded by relatively avascular areas (Maricq et al., 1980) (Fig. 5–3). With systemic lupus erythematosus, abnormal capillary loops are present and the subpapillary venous plexus may be more prominent; avascular areas are not present (Lee, 1985; Maricq et al., 1980). Patients with mixed connective tissue disease display bushy capillary formations more frequently than patients with scleroderma or lupus erythematosus (Granier et al., 1986). With rheumatoid arthritis, patients often have a normal nail-

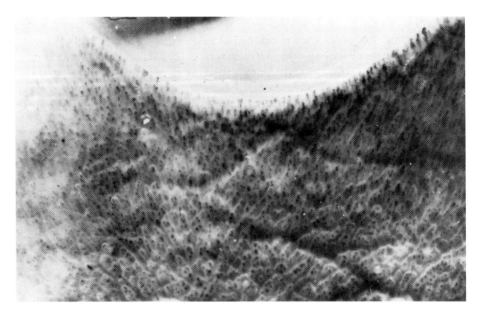

Fig. 5–2.   Capillary microscopy of the nailfold of a normal subject. Superficial capillaries are regularly spaced, hairpin loops aligned along the axis of the digits. *Source:* Maricq et al., 1980. Reprinted from *Arthritis and Rheumatism Journal,* © 1980. Used by permission of the American Rheumatism Association.

Fig. 5–3.   Capillary microscopy of the nailfold of a patient with scleroderma. Capillary loops are enlarged and deformed; relatively avascular areas surround the abnormal capillaries. *Source:* Maricq et al., 1980. Reprinted from *Arthritis and Rheumatism Journal,* © 1980. Used by permission of the American Rheumatism Association.

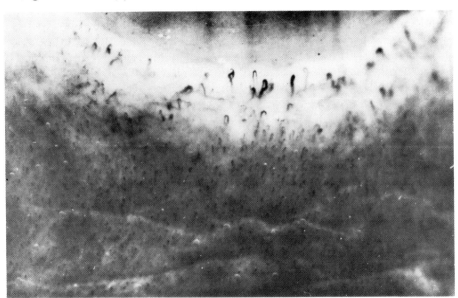

fold capillary pattern (Lee, 1985). Patients with primary Raynaud's disease usually have normal nailfold capillaries, but some have tortuous or dilated capillary loops; whether these patients will develop scleroderma later is unknown. Using a quantitative morphological analysis of the nailfold capillaries, Lefford and Edwards (1986) found normal capillary indices in three of nine patients with scleroderma, but they used rather stringent criteria for capillary selection. Other diseases, e.g., polymyositis, Sjögren's syndrome, Buerger's disease, and Behçet's disease, are occasionally associated with dystrophic, tortuous capillaries (Vayssairat et al., 1982b). With vibratory vasospastic disease, the number of capillary loops have been reported as signficiantly reduced (Vayssairat et al., 1982a).

Attempts have been made to classify the nailfold capillary findings. Maricq and co-workers (1976) used five classes:

Class I: normal or slightly dilated capillary loops only
Class II: definitely dilated loops confined to nailfold–distal phalanx
Class III: extremely dilated loops confined to nailfold–distal phalanx
Class IV: definitely dilated loops on nailfold–distal phalanx plus definitely dilated loops found on at least one other site
Class V: extremely dilated loops on nailfold–distal phalanx plus extremely dilated or definitely dilated loops found at another site

Lee and co-workers (1983) graded nailfold capillary changes according to overall avascularity (mild = one or two discrete areas of vascular deletion; moderate = more than two discrete areas; severe = large confluent avascular areas) and to vascular loop appearance as normal size, slightly enlarged, definitely enlarged, or extremely enlarged (giant loops).

These classifications probably add little to the diagnostic usefulness of the method but may help predict systemic involvement and prognosis of the connective tissue disease (Maricq et al., 1976). One study reported that decreased capillary density correlated with clinical findings of connective tissue disease, esophageal hypomotility, interstitial fibrosis on the chest x-ray film, organ system involvement, severity of vasospastic attacks, and the presence of autoantibodies and immune complexes in patients with Raynaud's phenomenon (Houtman et al., 1985). However, Lefford and Edwards (1986) found no relation between capillary morphology and clinical features of the diseases.

Capillary Red Blood Cell Flow Velocity

The capillary red blood cell flow velocity of the nailfold has been reported as decreased in primary Raynaud's disease, but this difference from normal subjects is less prominent at lower temperatures. With ice-cooled air blown on the nailfold, red blood cell flow in capillaries may stop in patients but only decrease in normal subejcts. Cessation of capillary flow is also seen in patients with scleroderma but not in those with Raynaud's phenomenon secondary to thromboangiitis obliterans (Mahler et al., 1977; Meier et al., 1978). Jacobs et al. (1987) also found a decrease in red blood cell velocity of capillaries before and after cold provocation in patients with primary Raynaud's disease or the secondary phenomenon; however, the capillaries were larger than in normal subjects, which could slow the red blood cell velocity.

Recovery Following Cold Exposure

The temperature or blood flow recovery time of digits after cold water exposure has been used for diagnosis and for studying the effect of treatment modalities in patients with Raynaud's phenomenon. One or both hands are immersed in ice or cool water for a given time. Ice water immersion of the hands seldom produces vasospastic attacks in the primary disease. The hands are dried, and the time to reach the preimmersion temperature of the digits is then determined with a thermocouple, thermistor, or skin temperature thermometer; blood flow may be measured using a variety of plethysmographic methods. After ice water immersion for 20 seconds, the time required for the fingers to return to preimmersion temperature usually exceeds 20 minutes in patients with Raynaud's phenomenon, whereas normal subjects regain the temperature within 5 to 20 minutes (Porter et al., 1975). The sensitivity and specificity of these tests for diagnosing primary Raynaud's disease or the secondary phenomenon due to a variety of diseases is low (Larouche and Theriault, 1987). Also, there is a large overlap between normal subjects and patients, and the test is not often reproducible. There has been no standardized temperature of the water or duration of hand immersion used by investigators. Water at ice temperatures to 20°C has been used, and immersion times have varied from 5 seconds to 2 minutes.

Arteriography

Arteriography of the digits, hand, and arm vessels usually demonstrates nonspecific findings that do not correlate with the diagnosis (Kent et al., 1976). Digital artery occlusions are seen in conjunction with most of the secondary causes of Raynaud's phenomenon and the severe cases of the primary disease (see Chap. 3). Ulnar and radial artery occlusions are often present with the connective tissue diseases, a finding that rules against the diagnosis of primary Raynaud's disease. Dabich and coworkers (1972) found organic arterial disease in 29 of 31 patients with scleroderma; digital artery occlusions were most common, but stenosis or occlusion of the ulnar artery was present in 16 patients and of the radial artery in two. Even patients without Raynaud's phenomenon showed diseased blood vessels. The arteriogram is most often normal in patients with the primary disease, but some patients with connective tissue disease or other secondary causes also have normal arteriograms (Jeune and Thivolet, 1978). Patients with rheumatoid arthritis frequently show digital artery occlusions when digital ischemia, subcutaneous nodules, and visceral involvement are present (Laws et al., 1963). The latter authors also considered multiple occlusive lesions distal to the palmar arch and irregular, tortuous digital arteries characteristic of polyarteritis nodosa, but in our experience this picture can be seen as well in conjunction with other secondary causes of Raynaud's phenomenon. The severity of arteriographic findings does not correlate with the response to treatment modalities such as sympathectomy (Kent et al., 1976). There is little indication for arteriography in Raynaud's phenomenon except to search for a source of suspected emboli.

Finger Total and Capillary Blood Flow

Total finger blood flow can be measured quantitatively by venous occlusion plethysmography, but this technique includes both capillary and arteriovenous shunt flow (see Chap. 1). Qualitative blood flow can be gauged by photoplethysmography and the laser–doppler. Capillary blood flow can be measured by the disappearance rate of a radioisotope from a local injection in the fingertip or after epicutaneous absorption of a radioisotope. Xenon 133 and Na[131]I have been used. The difference between capillary and total fingertip blood flow yields an estimate of the A-V shunt flow. Patients with primary and secondary Raynaud's phenomenon have, on average, smaller total and capillary fingertip blood flow in warm and cool environments than do normal subjects, but the overlap is too great for the measurement to be meaningful as a diagnostic test (Coffman and Cohen, 1971). In patients with scleroderma, Nilsen (1978) reported that the xenon 133 disappearance rate decreased underneath a small area of interdigital skin that was cooled, but no change or an increase occurred in normal subjects. This abnormality in skin blood flow occurred only at a temperature of 5°C; it is an interesting finding and needs to be confirmed.

Esophageal Motility

Esophageal motility is best measured by manometric or cineradiographic studies and has been used to diagnose secondary causes of Raynaud's phenomenon. Not all patients with motility abnormalities complain of heartburn, regurgitation, or dysphagia. Approximately 70 percent of patients with scleroderma have abnormal peristalsis of the lower two-thirds of the esophagus; the esophageal sphincter pressure may also be decreased (Turner et al., 1973; Weihrauch and Korting, 1982). Similar abnormalities occur in patients with mixed connective tissue disease and in some with lupus erythematosus (Gutierrez et al., 1982; Stevens et al., 1964; Tatelman and Keech, 1966). Some investigators have found a correlation of Raynaud's phenomenon with esophageal aperistalsis in these diseases as well as a correlation with the duration of scleroderma (Weihrauch and Korting, 1982). Significant pharyngeal and esophageal skeletal muscle dysfunction is an infrequent finding probably limited to polymyositis, although the upper one-third of the esophagus may be involved in the presence of mixed connective tissue disease (Gutierrez et al., 1982; Turner et al., 1973). Patients with rheumatoid arthritis have been reported to have normal motility studies (Tatelman and Keech, 1966). Some reports find no abnormalities in patients with primary Raynaud's disease (Weihrauch and Korting, 1982), but unfortunately other investigators have found lower esophageal abnormalities (Stevens et al., 1964). Whether this inconsistency means that the methodoloy is insensitive or that these patients will develop scleroderma in the future is unknown. Until this knowledge is obtained, the esophageal motility tests remain nondiagnostic.

Antinuclear Antibodies

The presence of antinuclear antibodies in a patient with Raynaud's phenomenon usually indicates that a systemic disease is present. The titer often correlates with the number of organ systems affected (Kallenberg et al., 1982a). A speckled pattern is most often indicative of scleroderma. With the CREST syndrome (calcinosis, Raynaud's phenomenon, esophageal involvement, sclerodactyly, telangiectasias), anticentromere antibodies are present in most of the patients (57–96 percent) and demonstrate a discrete, finely speckled pattern.

In 58 patients with Raynaud's phenomenon but no evidence of a definite underlying connective tissue disease, 31 percent who had the anticentromere antibody had more frequent digital telangiectasias, digital edema, increased immunoglobulins, low C4 values, and abnormal capillaries in their nailbeds than patients without the antibody (Sarkozi et al., 1987). The antibody therefore is indicative of an underlying disease, usually the CREST syndrome. Anticentromere antibodies are not common with other types of scleroderma. A homogeneous pattern of antinuclear antibodies with antibodies to desoxyribonucleic acid is often present in patients with systemic lupus erythematosus. Elderly patients may have an antinuclear antibody titer as high as 1:64 without systemic disease, whereas in younger patients it rarely exceeds 1:16. More specifics of antinuclear antibody tests are discussed in Chapter 6.

Erythrocyte Sedimentation Rate

The ESR is normal in patients with primary Raynaud's disease, whereas it is usually elevated in those with the connective tissue diseases. However, because one-third of patients with scleroderma may have a normal ESR and because elderly patients show an elevation, the test does not help in the diagnosis.

Platelet Products

Plasma β-thromboglobulin is a 36,000-dalton protein released from α-granules of platelets during activation. Measured by radioimmunoassay, its presence is an indication of the platelet aggregation that occurs in certain disease states. Seibold and co-workers (1985) found elevated levels of this platelet protein in 82 percent of patients with scleroderma. The level was not correlated with duration or extent of disease or with visceral involvement. In 19 patients with primary Raynaud's disease, β-thromboglobulin levels were not significantly different from those of normal control subjects. Seibold et al. also measured platelet factor 4, which has a half-life of 10 minutes. Because its levels were normal, artifactual platelet activation during phlebotomy or sample preparation was excluded. Kallenberg and co-workers (1982b) reported elevated β-thromboglobulin levels in 56 percent of patients with primary Raynaud's disease but no evidence of platelet activation (using the turbidometric technique). Zahavi and co-workers (1980) also found increased levels of β-thromboglobulin in 60 percent of patients with the primary disease as well as increased platelet aggregation in response to adenosine diphosphate. This difference in results in patients with the primary disease must be resolved before β-

thromboglobulin can be a useful diagnostic test for secondary Raynaud's phenomenon.

Finger Pulse Waves

Many investigators have reported pulse wave abnormalities measured on the fingers in patients with Raynaud's phenomenon. Pulse waves can be recorded by plethysmography, strain gauge technique, spectrometry, and laser methods. Sumner and Strandness (1972) described a "peaked pulse" with a rapid ascending limb and an anacrotic notch terminating in a sharp systolic peak; the dicrotic notch was high on the downstroke. They found a high incidence of this pulse abnormality in patients with cold sensitivity of unknown etiology and those with connective tissue diseases. The incidence of 44 percent was smaller in patients with primary Raynaud's disease. Pulse contours are not of diagnostic usefulness, as there is a large overlap between patients with primary Raynaud's disease and those with the secondary diseases that cause Raynaud's phenomenon even when vasospastic attacks have not been a manifestation.

Doppler Flowmeter Arterial Mapping

Arteries of the fingers can be traced with a doppler flowmeter, and this methodology has sometimes been used to study the effect of treatment modalities. However, absence of flow sounds does not differentiate obstruction from vasospasm of vessels. The day-to-day variation of digital arterial mapping is great. If all vessels can be demonstrated to be patent during a cold stimulus, patency not present previously during a cold stimulus could be attributed to a therapeutic modality preventing vasospasm.

SUMMARY

Raynaud's phenomenon is common in the general population, and the secondary diseases causing Raynaud's phenomenon do not approach this frequency; hence most patients must have the benign, primary disease. This fact must be considered during the work-up of patients. Few tests are indicated in patients who have well demarcated discoloration of the digits on cold exposure that is definitely espisodic in nature, who have no other symptoms, and whose physical examination is normal. Minimum laboratory work-up should include a complete blood count, urinalysis, chest radiography, and ESR. A more extensive work-up is necessary if any one of these tests is abnormal; further tests are also done in male patients, patients with onset of vasospastic attacks after age 40, and those with severe disease or trophic changes of the fingers. If the screening tests are normal, the patient can be assured that they likely have the benign, primary disease. Other tests with some degree of diagnostic usefulness are the determination of finger systolic pressure following a period of digital ischemia at progressively cooler local temperatures and nailfold capillary microscopy. However, these tests are cumbersome to perform, requiring specialized equipment, and they are not widely available. The former test does not differentiate primary from secondary disease, whereas the latter test may indicate the probability of the presence of a connective tissue disease.

Patients with Raynaud's phenomenon should be investigated for an underlying disease only when the history, physical examination, or routine laboratory tests indicate that one may be present. A complete work-up for all secondary causes would be expensive and not cost-effective. The initial examinations usually direct the diagnostic work-up into one channel. For example, a history of general fatigue, malaise, morning stiffness, achy joints, dysphagia, heartburn, fever, butterfly rash on the face, pleurisy, epilepsy, or muscle weakness, or a physical examination showing telangiectasias, tightening of the skin, rashes, discoloration of the eyelids, alopecia, or joint swelling, directs the diagnostic work-up toward the connective tissue diseases. However, a history of positional symptoms in the arms and positive maneuvers for a thoracic outlet syndrome indicate another diagnostic consideration. The various secondary causes and their diagnoses are discussed in Chapter 6.

REFERENCES

Allen EV, Brown GE: Raynaud's disease: a critical review of minimal requisites for diagnosis. *Am J Med Sci* 183:187, 1932.

Carter SA, Dean E, Kroeger EA: Apparent finger systolic pressures during cooling in patients with Raynaud's syndrome. *Circulation* 77:988, 1988.

Coffman JD: Evaluation of the patient with Raynaud's phenomenon. *Postgrad Med* 78:175, 1985.

Coffman JD, Cohen AS: Total and capillary fingertip blood flow in Raynaud's phenomenon. *N Engl J Med* 285:259, 1971.

Corbin DOC, Wood DA, Housley E: An evaluation of finger systolic-pressure response to local cooling in the diagnosis of primary Raynaud's phenomenon. *Clin Physiol* 5:383, 1985.

Dabich L, Bookstein JJ, Zweifler A, Zarafonetis CJD: Digital arteries in patients with scleroderma. *Arch Intern Med* 130:708, 1972.

Downs AR, Gaskell P, Morrow I, Munson CL: Assessment of arterial obstruction in vessels supplying the fingers by measurement of local blood pressures and the skin temperature response test—correlation with angiographic evidence. *Surgery* 77:530, 1975.

Granier F, Vayssairat M, Priollet P, Housset E: Nailfold capillary microscopy in mixed connective tissue disease. *Arthritis Rheum* 29:189, 1986.

Gutierrez F, Valenzuela JE, Ehresmann GR, Quismorio FP, Kitridori RC: Esophageal dysfunction in patients with mixed connective tissue diseases and systemic lupus erythematosus. *Dig Dis Sci* 27:592, 1982.

Hirai M: Arterial insufficiency of the hand evaluated by digital blood pressure and arteriographic findings. *Circulation* 58:902, 1978.

Hoare M, Miles C, Girvan R, Ramsden J, Needham T, Pardy B, Nicolaides A: The effect of local cooling on digital systolic pressure in patients with Raynaud's syndrome. *Br J Surg* 69(Suppl):S27, 1982.

Houtman PM, Kallenberg CGM, Wouda AA, The TH: Decreased nailfold capillary density in Raynaud's phenomenon: a reflection of immunologically mediated local and systemic vascular disease? *Ann Rheum Dis* 44:603, 1985.

Jacobs MJHM, Breslan PJ, Slaaf DW, Lemmens JAJ: Nomenclature of Raynaud's phenomenon: a capillary microscopy and hemorrheologic study. *Surgery* 101:136, 1987.

Jeune R, Thivolet J: Etude arteriographique de la main au cours de 52 phenomenes de Raynaud d'etiologie diverse. *Nouv Presse Med* 7:2619, 1978.

Kahlenbuhl B, Nielsen SL, Lassen NA: Closure of digital arteries in high vascular tone states as demonstrated by measurement of systolic blood pressure in fingers. *Scand J Clin Lab Invest* 37:71, 1977.

Kallenberg CGM, Pastoor GW, Wouda AA, The TH: Antinuclear antibodies in patients with Raynaud's phenomenon: clinical significance of anticentromere antibodies. *Ann Rheum Dis* 41:382, 1982a.

Kallenberg CGM, Vellenga E, Wouda AA, The TH: Platelet activation, fibrinolytic activity and circulating immune complexes in Raynaud's phenomenon. *J Rheumatol* 9:878, 1982b.

Kent SJS, Thomas ML, Browse NL: The value of arteriography of the hand in Raynaud's syndrome. *J Cardiovasc Surg* 17:72, 1976.

Larouche G-P, Theriault G: Validite de plethysmographie et du test de recuperation de la temperature digitale dans le diagnostic du phenomene de Raynaud primaire et professionnel. *Clin Invest Med* 10:96, 1987.

Laws JW, Lillie JG, Scott JC: Arteriographic appearances in rheumatoid arthritis and other disorders. *Br J Radiol* 36:477, 1963.

Lee P: Use of nailfold capillary microscopy in the diagnosis and assessment of systemic sclerosis and other connective tissue diseases. *Int Med Spec* 6:111, 1985.

Lee P, Leung FY-K, Alderdice C, Armstrong SK: Nailfold capillary microscopy in the connective tissue diseases: a semiquantitative assessment. *J Rheumatol* 10:930, 1983.

Lefford F, Edwards JCW: Nailfold capillary microscopy in connective tissue disease: a quantitative morphological analysis. *Ann Rheum Dis* 45:741, 1986.

Mahler F, Meier B, Frey R, Bollinger A, Anliker M: Reaction of red blood cell velocity in nailfold capillaries to local cold in patients with vasospastic disease. *Bibl Anat* 16:155, 1977.

Malamet R, Ettinger W, Wise RA, Wigley FM: Adaptability to cold provocation in Raynaud's phenomenon. *Clin Res* 32:701A, 1984.

Maricq HR, Spencer-Green G, LeRoy EC: Skin capillary abnormalities as indicators of organ involvement in scleroderma (systemic sclerosis), Raynaud's syndrome, and dermatomyositis. *Am J Med* 61:862, 1976.

Maricq HR, LeRoy EC, D'Angelo WA, Medsger TA, Rodnan GP, Sharp GG, Wolfe JF: Diagnostic potential of in vivo capillary microscopy in scleroderma and related disorders. *Arthritis Rheum* 23:183, 1980.

Meier B, Mahler F, Bollinger A: Blutflussgeschwingigkeit in Nagelfalzkapillaren bei Gesunden und Patienten mit vasospastischen und organischen akralen Durchblutungsstorungen. *Vasa* 7:194, 1978.

Nielsen SL: Raynaud phenomena and finger systolic pressure during cooling. *Scand J Clin Lab Invest* 38:765, 1978a.

Nielsen SL, Nobin BA, Hirai M, Eklof B: Raynaud's phenomenon in arterial obstructive disease of the hand demonstrated by locally provoked cooling. *Scand J Thorac Cardiovasc Surg* 12:105, 1978b.

Nilsen KH: Assessment of cold sensitivity in Raynaud's phenomenon associated with scleroderma. *Microvasc Res* 15:251, 1978.

Porter JM, Snider RL, Bardana EJ, Rosch J, Eidemiller LR: The diagnosis and treatment of Raynaud's phenomenon. *Surgery* 77:11, 1975.

Sarkozi J, Bookman AAM, Lee P, Keystone EC, Fritzler MJ: Significance of anticentromere antibody in idiopathic Raynaud's syndrome. *Am J Med* 83:893, 1987.

Seibold JR, Harris JN: Plasma β-thromboglobulin in the differential diagnosis of Raynaud's phenomenon. *J Rheumatol* 12:99, 1985.

Stevens MB, Hookman P, Siegel CI, Esterly JR, Shulman LE, Hendrix TR: Aperistalsis of the esophagus in patients with connective tissue disorders and Raynaud's phenomenon. *N Engl J Med* 270:1218, 1964.

Sumner DS, Strandness DE: An abnormal finger pulse associated with cold sensitivity. *Ann Surg* 175:294, 1972.

Tatelman M, Keech MK: Esophageal motility in systemic lupus erythematosus, rheumatoid arthritis, and scleroderma. *Radiology* 86:1041, 1966.

Turner R, Lipshutz W, Miller W, Rittenberg G, Schumacher HR, Cohen S: Esophageal dysfunction in collagen disease. *Am J Med Sci* 265:191, 1973.

Vayssairat M, Patri B, Guilmot JL, Housset E, Dubrisay J: La capillaroscopic dans la maladie des vibrations. *Nouv Presse Med* 11:3111, 1982a.

Vayssairat M, Priollet P, Golberg J, Housset E: Nailfold capillary microscopy as a diagnostic tool and in followup examination. *Arthritis Rheum* 25:597, 1982b.

Weihrauch TR, Korting GW: Manometric assessment of oesophageal involvement in progressive systemic sclerosis, morphoea, and Raynaud's disease. *Br J Dermatol* 107:325, 1982.

Zahavi J, Hamilton WAP, O'Reilly MJG, Leyton J, Cotton LT, Kakkar VV: Plasma exchange and platelet function in Raynaud's phenomenon. *Thromb Res* 19:85, 1980.

6

Secondary Causes of Raynaud's Phenomenon

The common secondary causes of Raynaud's phenomenon are drug therapy, connective tissue diseases, traumatic vasospastic disease, and the carpal tunnel and thoracic outlet syndromes (Table 6–1). In a tertiary referral hospital, the most frequent underlying cause is a connective tissue disease, and most of these patients have scleroderma (Coffman, personal observations; Blunt and Porter, 1981; Jeune and Thivolet, 1978). However, in a community practice, drug causes and the carpal tunnel and thoracic outlet syndromes are found more often. In foresting, brush cutting, and quarrying areas, traumatic vasospastic disease is common, and the hypothenar hammer syndrome is seen where meat processing plants are located. A thorough history and a physical examination usually uncover these secondary causes of Raynaud's phenomenon.

DRUGS

β-Adrenoceptor Blocking Drugs

Drugs that block the β-adrenoceptors are probably the most common pharmacological agents that induce Raynaud's phenomenon. Although β_2-adrenoceptors are considered to predominate in the peripheral circulation and β_1-adrenoceptors in the heart, both nonselective and cardioselective agents have been reported to induce vasospastic attacks. Most cardioselective agents, given in a large enough dose, are nonselective.

Incidence

Although some studies report an incidence of Raynaud's phenomenon (Vanden-Burg et al., 1984b) or cold extremities of only 4.1 percent, other investigators found a much higher incidence (as high as 40 percent) among hypertensive patients taking β-blocking drugs (Feleke et al., 1983; Marshall et al., 1976). One study found no increase in the prevalence of Raynaud's phenomenon in either men or women, although there was an increased incidence of cold extremities in men (Steiner et al., 1982). There is no apparent relation of the development of Raynaud's phenomenon in patients taking β-blocking drugs to age, sex, smoking, dose of drug, dura-

Table 6–1. Secondary Causes of Raynaud's Phenomenon

Drugs	Traumatic vasospastic disease
β-Adrenoceptor blocking agents	Carpal tunnel syndrome
Ergot preparations	Thoracic outlet syndrome
Methysergide	Hypothenar hammer syndrome
Vinblastine and bleomycin	Obstructive arterial disease
Nitroglycerin	Arteriosclerosis obliterans
Amphetamines	Thromboangiitis obliterans
Imipramine	Arterial emboli
Bromocriptine and clonidine	Reflex sympathetic dystrophy
Cyclosporin	Blood abnormalities
Oral contraceptives	Polycythemia
Connective tissue diseases	Cryoproteinemias
Scleroderma	Cold agglutinins
Systemic lupus erythematosus	Vinyl chloride disease
Polymyositis and dermatomyositis	Neoplasms
Rheumatoid arthritis and Sjögren's	Hypothyroidism
syndrome	Hepatitis B antigenemia
Mixed connective tissue diseases	Unknown causes and vasculitis
Psoriasis and Raynaud's phenomenon	Intraarterial injections
Raynaud's phenomenon and primary pulmonary	Arteriovenous fistula
hypertension	Renal disease

tion of treatment, use of vibratory tools, or arteriosclerosis obliterans (Feleke et al., 1983; Marshall et al., 1976). Severe digital ischemia has developed in rare patients (Frohlich et al., 1969; Vale and Jefferys, 1978), but usually the symptoms do not require withdrawal of the drug (Zacharias, 1976).

Other Antihypertensive Agents

In some studies many patients with hypertension have complained of cold extremities before drug therapy, whereas in other studies the incidence has been low. Marshall and co-workers (1976) found that only 1 of 21 patients on methyldopa developed Raynaud's phenomenon, whereas 41 percent of patients on β-blocking drugs were afflicted. Feleke and co-workers (1983) reported that 18 percent of patients on diuretics developed cold extremities, whereas the incidence was 40 percent among those on β-blocking agents, a statistically significant difference. VandenBurg and co-workers (1984a) discovered cold extremities in only 0.4 percent of patients on methyldopa, 0.2 percent of patients on other drugs, and 4.1 percent of patients on β-blockers. In the Medical Research Council Working Party study on hypertension (1981), there was a significant increase in the incidence of Raynaud's phenomenon in both sexes on propranolol, which led to withdrawal from treatment. This group was compared to patients treated with a diuretic or placebo. The incidence was 5.4 percent of men and 5.6 percent of women on propranolol but less than 0.5 percent in the other groups. Forty percent of patients developed Raynaud's phenomenon within 3 months and 70 percent by 1 year of treatment. Therefore other antihypertensive agents cannot be implicated.

Nonselective versus Cardioselective β-Blockers

Vasospastic attacks and cold extremities have developed in patients taking propranolol, alprenolol, atenolol, oxyprenolol, and metoprolol. Some investigators have found a lesser incidence of the phenomenon with the cardioselective agents, but others have not. Nielsen and Nielsen (1981) reported a greater decrease in finger systolic pressure during finger cooling with propranolol (120–240 mg daily) than with metoprolol (100–150 mg daily) or a thiazide diuretic. McSorley and Warren (1978) found a greater decrease in skin temperature and in skin and muscle blood flow with propranolol (80 mg) compared to metoprolol (100 mg) in single doses. Lenders and colleagues (1986) measured the recovery of finger skin temperature after hand immersion in 16°C water for 5 minutes in normal subjects during treatment with propranolol, atenolol, pindolol, or acebutolol. They found a quicker recovery of skin temperature after propranolol (80 mg three times a day) and no difference in recovery times among the other three drugs. Wollersheim and co-workers (1987), using the same technique, also found no difference between nonselective and selective β-blocking drugs in patients with hypertension. Thus there is conflicting evidence that cardioselective agents may have less effect on skin blood flow than the nonselective drugs.

β-Blocking Drugs with Intrinsic Sympathetic Activity

β-Blocking drugs with intrinsic sympathetic activity have also been studied, and the results have been conflicting. Feleke and co-workers (1983) reported no difference in symptoms in patients on pindolol compared to other β-blocking agents. Eliasson and co-workers (1982) found that six of ten patients who developed vasospastic symptoms with metoprolol reported fewer symptoms when given pindolol. However, the patients did not show an improvement in skin temperature after hand exposure to 15°C water for 15 minutes with pindolol compared to that seen with metoprolol. Eliasson and co-workers (1979) treated patients who developed vasospastic symptoms on β-blocking drugs with a β-receptor-stimulating drug, terbutaline, for 3 weeks. No change in skin temperature after cool water immersion of the hand occurred with terbutaline treatment.

β- and α-Adrenoceptor Blocking Drugs

Agents with both β- and α-adrenoceptor blocking activity have also been studied, again with variable results. Heck and co-investigators (1981) reported that labetalol, a drug with both β- and α-adrenoceptor blocking activity, increased finger blood flow in patients with essential hypertension during acute or chronic administration. Erb and Plachetka (1985) found no difference in the digital plethysmogram and no decrease in hand temperature with smoking between labetalol and propranolol in six subjects. Steiner and co-workers (1979) studied 14 patients with hypertension and Raynaud's phenomenon in a double-blind crossover study of propranolol (160 mg) and labetalol (600 mg). They found no significant differences between the two drugs in terms of finger temperature or symptoms. In open trials, Bolli and co-workers (1977) and Eliasson and colleagues (1984) changed patients who developed vasospastic symptoms during β-adrenoceptor blockade to labetalol and reported symptomatic improvement; the former investigators also found decreased temperature sensitivity as determined by finger systolic pressure during local cooling with labetalol. Van der Veur and co-workers (1985) compared atenolol, propranolol, and labetalol in 12 patients with hypertension in a single-blind, crossover study; peripheral symptoms were similar with all three drugs, but finger pulses during cooling were better preserved with labetalol. Thus the evidence is slim that labetalol is a better choice than β-adrenoceptor blocking agents in hypertensive patients to avoid digital vasospastic side effects.

β-Blocking Drugs in Patients with Raynaud's Phenomenon

β-Adrenoceptor blocking agents may be needed for treatment of coronary artery. disease in patients who already have Raynaud's phenomenon. Steiner and co-workers (1979) administered propranolol (160 mg) or labetalol (600 mg) daily to 14 hypertensive patients with Raynaud's phenomenon in a double-blind crossover study and found no differences in finger temperatures or symptoms by diary compared to a placebo period for either drug. Holti (1982) studied 12 patients with hypertension and Raynaud's phenomenon in a double-blind, crossover study of propranolol (160 mg of a long-acting preparation daily) and acebutolol (400 mg daily), a cardioselective agent. From various indirect tests of the digital circulation, Holti concluded that acebutolol caused less impairment of the peripheral circulation than did propranolol in these patients. Coffman and Rasmussen (1985) studied the effect of propranolol (80 mg daily) and metoprolol (100 mg daily) in a double-blind, crossover study in 16 nonhypertensive patients with Raynaud's phenomenon (14 patients with primary Raynaud's disease). There were no significant changes in total fingertip blood flow, capillary blood flow, or finger systolic pressure in a warm or cool environment during treatment with either drug compared with

Fig. 6–1. Total fingertip blood flow in a warm and cool environment in 16 patients with Raynaud's phenomenon during treatment with placebo, metoprolol, and propranolol. Data are means ± SEM. There were no significant differences between drug and placebo periods or between the two drug periods in the warm or the cool room. *Source:* Coffman and Rasmussen (1985).

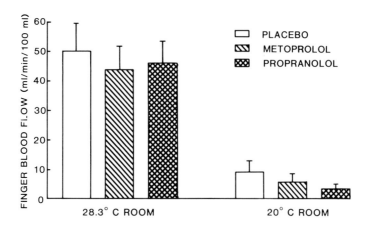

Table 6-2. Frequency of Vasospastic Attacks and Patients' Subjective Evaluation during Placebo or β-Adrenoceptor Blocking Drug Administration

Drug	Vasospastic attacks/2 weeks	Subjective evaluation
Placebo	15.3 ± 4.0	2.0 ± 0.1
Metroprolol	14.3 ± 3.8	2.4 ± 0.3
Placebo	15.8 ± 5.3	2.1 ± 0.3
Propranolol	14.5 ± 4.0	2.4 ± 0.2

Data are mean $\pm$ SE. There were no significant differences between the four 2-week periods. Subjective evaluation: 1 = worse; 2 = unchanged; 3 = 25 to 50% improved; 4 = 50 to 75% improved; 5 = 75 to 100% improved.

the placebo period (Fig. 6-1). There were also no significant changes in the number of vasospastic attacks or the patients' overall evaluation of their condition while they were receiving the drugs (Table 6-2). It can be concluded that the presence of Raynaud's phenomenon is not a contraindication to the use of β-adrenoceptor blocking drugs.

Pathophysiology
How β-adrenoceptor blocking agents induce Raynaud's phenomenon is unknown. β-Adrenoceptors have been shown to be present in the arteriovenous (A-V) anastomoses of the finger (Cohen and Coffman, 1981). They are responsive only to humoral agents and not to neurogenic stimulation, but they could be involved in the development of Raynaud's phenomenon. Unopposed α-adrenoceptor vasoconstrictor activity is another possible mechanism, and increased sensitivity to α-adrenoceptor stimulation in peripheral vessels has been shown during β-adrenoceptor blockade (White and Udwadia, 1975). It has been postulated that the decrease in cardiac output or blood volume produced by β-adrenoceptor blockade induces a reflex vasoconstriction of peripheral vessels leading to the vasospastic phenomenon. Also, an increased reflex sympathetic vasoconstriction caused by the central cardiovascular depressant effects of β-adrenoceptor blockade has been suggested, which could explain why cardioselective agents also induce Raynaud's phenomenon. Almost all studies reporting the development of Raynaud's phenomenon or cold extremities with these drugs have been in hypertensive patients. Nielsen and co-workers (1981) have demonstrated that digital arterial tone during cooling is significantly greater among hypertensive patients than among normotensive controls. Therefore hypertensive patients may be more apt to develop this side effect of β-adrenoceptor blockade. Vasospastic phenomena do occur in nonhypertensive patients treated with these drugs; 8 of 21 patients reported by Eliasson and co-workers (1979) did not have high blood pressure.

Summary
Raynaud's phenomenon or cold extremities may occur in patients treated with β-adrenoceptor blocking agents, whether cardioselective or nonselective. The sexes are equally affected, in contrast to the high prevalence of female patients with primary Raynaud's disease. Substitution of a drug with intrinsic sympathomimetic β-

adrenoceptor or with α-adrenoceptor blocking activity has not been clearly shown to be beneficial. Approximately 5 percent of hypertensive patients required withdrawal of β-adrenoceptor blocking drugs or reduction of the dose because of Raynaud's phenomenon. The presence of Raynaud's phenomenon is not a contraindication to the use of β-adrenoceptor blocking drugs in the normotensive or hypertensive population.

Ergot Preparations

Ergot has long been known to produce intense vasospasm and is more likely to induce prolonged ischemia of the digits than episodic Raynaud's phenomenon. Epidemics of ergot intoxication appeared in Europe from the Middle Ages until three decades ago and were due to eating foods made from rye contaminated with the fungus *Claviceps purpurea*. The most common cause now, however, is the use of ergotamine preparations for the treatment of migraine headaches.

Pathophysiology
Ergotamine induces vasoconstriction by stimulating the α-adrenoceptors to which the drug is tightly bound (Innes, 1962). In dog arteries ergotamine may act through serotonergic receptors (Muller-Schweinitzer, 1976), but this mechanism has not been demonstrated in humans. The venoconstrictor effect on human superficial veins by ergot alkaloids is blocked by phentolamine, indicating an α-adrenergic action (Aellig, 1976). Using digital plethysmography in humans, Bluntschli and Goetz (1948) demonstrated transient vasodilatation followed by vasoconstriction with intravenous ergotamine. However, in sympathectomized limbs only vasoconstriction occurred, indicating that the sympatholytic action is via the central nervous system.

Pathology
Both Kaunitz (1932) and Lewis (1935) studied the effect of ergot feeding or ergotamine systemic injections on the combs of fowl. Kaunitz reported intimal proliferation and thromboses of blood vessels. Lewis demonstrated that the drug constricts the arteries and damages the endothelium, leading to stasis and thrombosis, which results in necrosis. The vasoconstriction was unrelieved by body or local warming. In man proliferation of the endothelium, thrombosis, hyaline degeneration, and fibrosis of the vascular wall have been described in severe cases.

Dose, Incidence, Sex
Ergotamine toxicity is usually due to excessive doses of the drug, most commonly from suppositories but also from oral ingestion. Symptoms usually have occurred in patients whose dosage exceeded 10 mg of ergotamine per week, although symptoms have been reported with lesser doses (Cameron and French, 1960). The incidence of toxicity is 0.01 percent of patients using the drug, and women have been affected more than men, in a ratio of 5:1. Various factors have been said to increase the susceptibility to toxicity, but they are poorly documented. Propranolol, which also can induce Raynaud's phenomenon, was reported as a possible complicating

factor in one woman who developed vasospasm after 10 mg of ergotamine (Greenberg and Hallett, 1982). The lower extremities have been most often affected, but the upper extremities may be the only involvement. Usually the extremities are symmetrically involved, but it is variable. Vasospasm of the carotid, axillary, renal, coronary, ophthalmic, and splanchnic vessels (Greene et al., 1977) has also occurred.

Clinical Picture

The patient usually presents with painful, cold, often discolored extremities, although occasional patients complain only of intermittent claudication. Rarely, patients complain of an intense burning pain that has been called St. Anthony's fire (Cameron and French, 1960). Often no pulses except the carotid and femoral pulses are palpable, and the extremities are cold and cyanotic. Patients have developed gangrene requiring amputation of digits or extremities.

Diagnosis

A history of ergotamine use and the physical examination may be all that is necessary for the diagnosis. In other patients arteriography may be helpful. The arteriogram usually shows uniformly smooth tapering of the large and medium-sized arteries, with the vessels sometimes disappearing at the forearm or calf level. Collateral vessels are present in some cases, and thrombus formation is found occasionally (Bagby and Cooper, 1972; Herlache et al., 1973; Husted et al., 1978). However, atypical pictures may be seen. Kempczinski and co-workers (1976) reported a patient with a severe stenosis of the superficial femoral artery in the adductor canal, which was irregular and typical of arteriosclerosis obliterans. On withdrawal of the ergotamine, a follow-up arteriogram showed normal vasculature.

If systolic pressures are measured at the ankle level, they are usually decreased. In fact, Dige-Petersen and colleagues (1977) found low-normal or abnormal systolic pressures at the ankle and first toe in 32 patients who had been taking ergotamine for more than 1 year; only one patient was symptomatic. In 13 patients who stopped the drug, the systolic pressure rose significantly and was normal within 9 days.

Treatment

A large variety of drugs have been used to treat ergotamine vasospasm. Most reports of successful drug therapy, however, involve only one or two patients. Nifedipine (Dagher et al., 1985; Kemerer et al., 1984), nitroprusside (Carliner et al., 1974; Dierckx et al., 1986; Husted et al., 1978; O'Dell et al., 1977), streptokinase (Brismar et al., 1977), nitroglycerin (Husum et al., 1979; Tfelt-Hansen et al., 1982), prazosin (Cobaugh, 1980), hydralazine (Carliner et al., 1974), captopril (Zimran et al., 1984), phenoxybenzamine (Greenberg and Hallett, 1982; Hessov et al., 1972), tolazoline (Cameron and French, 1960; Greenberg and Hallett, 1982; Shifrin et al., 1980), hydergine (Cameron and French, 1960), sodium nicotinate (Young and Humphries, 1961), papaverine (Hessov et al., 1972), phentolamine, and chlorpromazine have all been recommended. In many of these cases the drug was not given until several days after ergotamine was stopped; it is therefore difficult to evalute their effectiveness, as ergotamine vasospasm often reverses within a few days. For all the reports of successful drug therapy, there are others that are contradictory. The large number of drugs that have been tried speaks to the fact that such therapy is often unsuccessful. Sympathetic blocks have been used mostly without success (Dagher et al., 1985; Husted et al., 1978; Kemerer et al., 1984; Shifrin et al., 1980), and periarterial stripping has been recommended (Young and Humphries, 1961). Interruption of the sympathetic nerves is not logical, as sympathectomized limbs are more susceptible to the vasoconstrictor action of ergotamine and because the drug does not act via the sympathetic nervous system. Shifrin and co-workers (1980) reported two patients in whom balloon-tipped catheter dilatation produced immediate and sustained release of ergotamine-induced vasospasm after unsuccessful sympathetic blockade or drug therapy. No further reports of this therapy have been published.

In patients who do not appear to have limb-threatening vasospasm, conservative therapy is the best course, as the vasospasm usually dissipates within 3 days after the ergotamine is stopped. Anticoagulation with heparin or dextran infusions is advisable to prevent thromboses. In patients with limb- or digit-threatening vasospasm, intraarterial or intravenous nitroprusside alone or with oral nifedipine is apparently the most successful of the drug therapies.

Methysergide

Methysergide is a congener of lysergic acid diethylamide (LSD) and an ergot derivative that has some vasoconstrictor activity. It is a serotonin antagonist but also has some agonist activity. It potentiates the pressor action of norepinephrine, epinephrine, and nicotine. Several cases of ischemia of the upper and lower extremity have occurred during the use of methysergide for migraine headaches. The incidence of this complication has been estimated at 3 percent and may occur with small (1 mg) or large doses (Graham, 1964). Combination use with ergotamine preparations has been reported to cause severe vasoconstriction in some patients (Johnson, 1966). Patients present with cold, numb extremities and decreased or absent pulses. Ameli and co-workers (1977) described one patient who demonstrated a reversible occlusion of the brachial artery proved by angiography. Treatment consists of withdrawal of the drug and use of vasodilating agents when necessary as outlined under ergotamine toxicity treatment.

Vinblastine and Bleomycin

Incidence and Pathophysiology
Vinblastine and bleomycin therapy for testicular carcinomas (Chernicoff, 1978; Teutsch et al., 1977; Vogelzang et al., 1981), lymphomas (Elomaa et al., 1984), and head or neck tumors (Kukla et al., 1982) has been reported to induce Raynaud's phenomenon or digital ischemia in 2.6 percent (Scheulen and Schmidt, 1982) to 37 percent (Vogelzang et al., 1981) of patients. It is not known if one or both of these agents are of etiological importance. Rothberg (1978) reported a patient in whom

Raynaud's phenomenon developed 22 months after bleomycin therapy was discontinued; vinblastine, which the patient was still receiving, was implicated. However, Raynaud's phenomenon may develop after treatment with these drugs is stopped (Soble, 1978). Vinblastine can cause neuropathy and therefore may interfere with the autonomic nervous system. Bleomycin causes cutaneous toxicity manifested by plaques, nodules, and bands on the hands as well as linear hyperpigmentation on the trunk in some patients; it has also (rarely) induced sclerodermatous skin changes (Cohen et al., 1973).

Clinical Picture

Symptoms appear after about 10 months of therapy. There is no apparent relation to age, histological subtype of the tumor, presence of α-fetoprotein or chorionic gonadotropin, dose of drugs, cutaneous or neurotoxicity, or renal dysfunction after treatment (Vogelzang et al., 1981). There is a higher incidence in patients who smoke cigarettes. The vasospastic attacks may be mild to severe, with digital gangrene developing in a few patients (Elomaa et al., 1984). Arteriograms have shown diffuse digital artery narrowing or multiple digital and palmar arterial occlusions (Grau et al., 1983; Vogelzang et al., 1981). Cerebrovascular accidents have also been reported in patients with underlying cardiovascular disease (Kukla et al., 1982).

Prognosis

After treatment with the chemotherapeutic agents is complete, patients may show marked improvement in their vasospastic manifestations (Teutsch et al., 1977). Some patients, however, continue to have Raynaud's phenomenon. There is an indication, although not proved, that concomitant therapy with prednisone during chemotherapy may decrease the incidence of Raynaud's phenomenon (Scheulen and Schmidt, 1982). In our experience, Raynaud's phenomenon is common in patients being treated with vinblastine and bleomycin for testicular tumors, and symptoms often persist following treatment.

Nitroglycerin

Workers in nitroglycerin and munitions factories may develop vasospasm during their weekends off or vacations. It is postulated that vasoconstriction occurs following withdrawal from chronic exposure to the vasodilator. The incidence has been estimated at 5 percent. Most patients develop angina pectoris, although one patient was reported to have digital artery vasospasm (Lange et al., 1972).

Amphetamines

One case of diffuse arterial spasm has been described after ingestion of 4-bromo-2,5-dimethoxyamphetamine (Bower et al., 1983). Arteriography showed vasoconstriction of the brachial and distal arteries. Treatment with intravenous nitroprusside was successful.

Imipramine

A 37-year-old woman developed Raynaud's phenomenon within 10 days of taking imipramine 150 mg daily (Appelbaum and Kapoor, 1983). The syndrome disappeared 4 months after stopping the drug but reappeared within 5 days of readministration at half the dose. This same patient developed vasospastic episodes with amitriptyline later. The mechanism of action is unknown; tricyclic antidepressants inhibit norepinephrine reuptake and increase norepinephrine levels, but they are also antagonists of α_1-adrenergic activity.

Bromocriptine and Clonidine

Bromocriptine mesylate is an ergot derivative with dopamine agonist activity. It is used to treat Parkinson's disease, hyperprolactinemia, and acromegaly. Raynaud's phenomenon may occur with its use, probably due to stimulation of the α-adrenoceptors.

Clonidine is an imidazoline derivative used to treat hypertension. It rarely causes Raynaud's phenomenon. It does stimulate peripheral α-adrenoceptors, but its main antihypertensive action is stimulating central α-adrenoceptors, resulting in decreased sympathetic outflow to peripheral vessels.

We have seen several cases of Raynaud's phenomenon during bromocriptine therapy but only one during clonidine treatment. The vasospastic attacks were mild and did not necessitate interruption of therapy.

Cyclosporin

Deray and co-workers (1986) described two patients who developed Raynaud's phenomenon during treatment with cyclosporin. In one of the patients the vasospastic attacks ceased and reappeared with cessation and then resumption of the drug therapy. Evidently, cyclosporin did not change plasma and urinary catecholamine levels, and it inhibited the renin-angiotensin system, which rules against a sympathetic or angiotensin mechanism. There was a decrease in 6-keto-prostaglandin(PG) F_1 urinary excretion (6-keto-PGF_1 is a metabolite of the potent vasodilator prostacyclin), which could help explain the adverse vascular effect.

Oral Contraceptives

Oral contraceptives have been mentioned as a cause of Raynaud's phenomenon or digital artery thromboses and local gangrene (Birnstingl, 1971) but little substantiation exists in the literature. Bole and co-workers (1969) reported eight women who developed rheumatic symptoms and had positive antinuclear antibodies. Three of these patients had Raynaud's phenomenon, but only one developed it during contraceptive therapy after 26 months. One patient had lupus erythematosus. Vasospastic attacks were said to be increased during the hormonal therapy. There is no evidence that Raynaud's phenomenon occurs with increased frequency in women who take oral contraceptives compared to nonusers. We have not been impressed that Raynaud's phenomenon is exacerbated by oral contraceptives or improved by their discontinuation.

CONNECTIVE TISSUE DISEASES

Scleroderma

Incidence, Sex, Early Clinical Picture
Vasospastic attacks typical of Raynaud's phenomenon or persistent vasospasm manifested by cyanosis during cold exposure occurs in 90 percent of patients with scleroderma, or systemic sclerosis (Tuffanelli and Winkelmann, 1961). It is the presenting symptom in almost 50 percent of patients. Vasospastic attacks are by definition part of the CREST syndrome (Thibierge and Weissenbach, 1911), a usually but not always less severe form of scleroderma. (CREST = subcutaneous calcification, Raynaud's phenomenon, esophageal dysfunction, sclerodermatous skin thickening, and telangiectasias.) We have also seen Raynaud's phenomenon in the localized form of scleroderma, termed scleroderma morphea.

Patients who have Raynaud's phenomenon with other systemic complaints, physical findings suggestive of other diseases, or abnormal laboratory tests should not be assured they have the benign form of primary Raynaud's disease (see Chap. 5). In the early stages, Raynaud's phenomenon may be the only manifestation of scleroderma; physical findings may be absent and laboratory tests normal. Scleroderma, like primary Raynaud's disease, occurs more often in female patients but the female/male ratio is about 3:1 (Tuffanelli and Winkelmann, 1961). Abnormalities of lower esophageal motility lead to a high incidence of heartburn or difficulty swallowing in patients with scleroderma. Lower esophageal motor abnormalities have also been described with primary Raynaud's disease, but it is not clear that these patients were not in the early stages of scleroderma (Hostein et al., 1985). Patients with early disease may also complain of generalized arthralgias or even arthritis.

CREST Syndrome
With the CREST syndrome, patients have vasospastic attacks of the fingers and often the toes. Telangiectasias are found most commonly on the fingers, eyelids, malar areas, mucous membranes of the mouth (especially the tongue), and the skin of the anterior and posterior chest. Heartburn and dysphagia are common complaints, but abnormal esophageal motility may be found only by barium swallow or manometry. There is a tightening or thickening of the skin of the extremities and face; the upper and lower extremities may have subcutaneous edema. Subcutaneous calcifications can often be palpated on the fingers or around the elbows, knees, or ankles, or they may appear as elevated indurated plaques. The subcutaneous calcifications may ulcerate and exude a whitish, thick material; infections of the areas are common. The ulcerations are painful and may not heal until the calcium deposition drains or is surgically removed. Digital ulcerations from ischemia of the fingertips is common with scleroderma but may also be caused by the sub-

cutaneous diffuse or localized calcifications. Radiographs of the hands may disclose this calcification when it is not clinically apparent. With nonhealing ulcers, radiographs should always be obtained.

Late Clinical Picture

The clinical picture in the more advanced cases of scleroderma is usually diagnostic. Symptoms include Raynaud's phenomenon, often with painful digital ulcerations, sclerodactyly, heartburn, dysphagia, arthralgias or arthritis, and dyspnea on exertion due to pulmonary involvement. Physical findings are characteristic. Because of the tightening of the facial skin with recession of the lips, the gums are often visible (Fig. 6-2). This facial deformity causes many scleroderma patients to have a strong resemblance to each other. One of the early signs of facial skin tightening is the inability to open the mouth to the normal 5 cm. Sclerodactyly is a claw finger deformity of the hands that is caused by thickened skin and contracture of the phalangeal joints (Fig. 6-3). Ulcers usually form at the distal fingertips or around the nail beds. Telangiectasias may be sparse or may cover the malar area and fingers. Esophageal strictures may develop, leading to vomiting or aspiration pneumonitis. Lung examination may be normal or reveal fine, crackly rales at the bases. Hypertension may occur due to renal involvement.

Sequestration of the terminal phalanges or the development of gangrene may lead to autoamputation, or it may necessitate surgical amputation. Sclerodactyly cannot be considered diagnostic of scleroderma, as only 3 of 71 patients with sclerodactyly developed the systemic disease when followed for an average of 10 years (Farmer et al., 1961).

Fig. 6-2. Typical facies of a woman with scleroderma. Facial skin tightening causes lip retraction, baring the gums and smoothing the forehead skin. Telangiectasias are present on the malar areas and the nose.

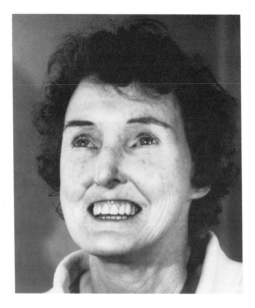

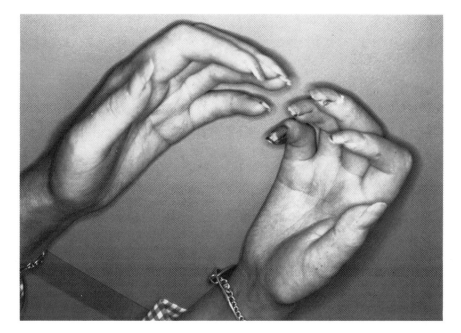

Fig. 6-3. Sclerodactyly of the hands of a patient with scleroderma. The skin on the fingers is tight, shiny, and indurated. The fingers are retracted in the flexed position because of the skin tightening. There is loss of subcutaneous tissue on the distal fingers, and a small ulceration is present on the third finger of the hand in the left side of the picture.

Laboratory Studies

Laboratory examinations are sometimes normal even with far-advanced disease. The erythrocyte sedimentation rate (ESR) is normal in one-third of patients. The complete blood count and urinalysis are often normal. Antinuclear antibodies are usually present in the advanced stages of the disease and are often of the speckled pattern (Tan et al., 1980). Antinuclear antibody is directed against a soluble nuclear antigen called SCL-70, nucleolar RNA, or the centromere of chromosomes. The CREST syndrome usually has an anticentromere antibody (Fritzler and Kinsella, 1980), whereas systemic sclerosis has a high incidence of anti-SCL-70 and anti-nucleolar antibodies. Barium swallow examination or esophageal manometry reveals the esophageal dysfunction, which is limited to the lower smooth muscle portion of the esophagus. Chest radiographs may show linear streaks of fibrosis in the basal areas of the lungs. Wide-field microscopic examination of the nail beds reveals sparse, dilated, convoluted capillaries and avascular areas (see Chap. 5).

Diagnosis

The American Rheumatism Association has recommended preliminary criteria for the diagnosis of scleroderma (Masi and Rodman, 1980) (Table 6-3). A useful diagnostic classification has been proposed by LeRoy and colleagues (1988). They divided scleroderma into two subsets: diffuse cutaneous scleroderma and limited

Table 6–3.   Preliminary Criteria for Classification of Scleroderma[a]

Major criterion
Scleroderma skin changes proximal to acral parts
Minor criteria
Sclerodactyly
Digital pitting scars
Bibasilar pulmonary fibrosis

[a]The presence of either the major criterion or two or more of the minor criteria determines the diagnosis. *Source:* Masi and Rodnan (1980).

scleroderma. The former is characterized by diffuse skin changes soon after the onset of Raynaud's phenomenon; tendon friction rubs; early lung, kidney, gastrointestinal, or myocardial involvement; nailfold capillary destruction; antitopoisomerase antibodies in 30 percent of patients; and an absence of anticentromere antibodies. Limited scleroderma is characterized by Raynaud's phenomenon that has been present for years; limited skin involvement of acral parts, if any; a late incidence of pulmonary hypertension with or without lung disease, trigeminal neuralgia, subcutaneous calcifications, and telangiectasia; a high incidence of anticentromere antibody; and dilated nailfold capillary loops.

Etiology and Pathology
The etiology of scleroderma is unknown; controversy continues about whether it is a disease of collagen tissue or a vascular disease. Pathology studies of the skin reveal edema and chronic inflammatory cells early, although homogeneous, acellular deposits of collagen in indistinct bundles are often present. There is a loss of capillaries, and arterioles may show hyalinization. Internal organs often show extensive fibrotic changes.

Pathophysiology
There is evidence that Raynaud's phenomenon associated with scleroderma is produced by abnormalities of the vessel wall but also that there may be sympathetic nervous system dysfunction. The walls of small arteries and arterioles are often thickened; and on electron microscopy, thickening and reduplication of basement membranes are apparent. As the disease progresses, the blood vessels are entrapped in nondistensible fibrous tissue. Tissue pressures of up to 320 mm H_2O were present in patients compared to the upper limit of 54 mm H_2O in normal subjects in a study by Sodeman and Burch (1939). However, sclerodermatous skin does not always have decreased blood flow (Coffman, 1970). When measured by the disappearance rate of a radioisotope, no significant difference in forearm skin or subcutaneous blood flow was found between patients and normal subjects (Fig. 6-4). The forearm skin was clinically thickened in seven of the eight patients studied. The averages for cutaneous blood flow in the foreheads and fingertips of patients were significantly smaller than in normal subjects, but normal disappearance rates were sometimes obtained from obviously involved skin in these areas as well. The normal forearm cutaneous blood flow was confirmed by another group of investigators (LeRoy et al., 1971). These studies indicate that a decrease in nutritional blood flow is not the primary etiological factor for scleroderma.

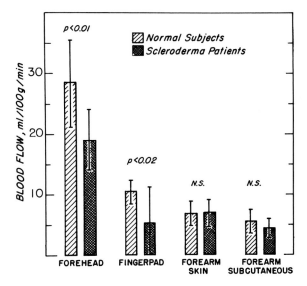

Fig. 6–4. Blood flow was measured in various skin areas and in forearm subcutaneous tissue of patients with scleroderma and normal subjects by the disappearance rate of a radioisotope from a local depot. Mean blood flows ± standard deviations are shown. Forearm skin and subcutaneous tissue were clinically involved in all but one patient, but there was no significant difference in skin or subcutaneous blood flow between patients and normal subjects. The averages for cutaneous blood flow in the foreheads and fingertips of patients were significantly decreased compared to normal subjects. *Source:* Coffman (1970).

Increased sympathetic activity has been postulated as the cause of the vasospastic attacks of scleroderma (Jablonska, 1965), but it is more likely that there is hypoactivity. Fries (1969) measured electrical skin resistance, an index of sympathetic activity, in 33 patients with scleroderma, 15 patients with Raynaud's phenomenon suspected of having scleroderma, and normal subjects. There was no evidence of increased activity in the patients, and decreased activity was found in their fingertips. Also, forehead skin blood flow in patients with scleroderma does not show an increased response to sympathetic stimulation compared to that in normal subjects (Coffman, 1970). Sapira and co-workers (1972) found venous plasma and urinary catecholamine levels to be no higher in patients with Raynaud's phenomenon due to scleroderma than in a control group of other hospitalized patients.

Systemic Lupus Erythematosus

Incidence, Sex, Age

Systemic lupus erythematosus (SLE) is a multisystem disorder that affects skin, blood vessels, kidney, brain, synovial and serous membranes, and blood constituents. It occurs predominantly in women in the 20- to 40-year-old age group; the incidence is higher in Blacks than Caucasians. Raynaud's phenomenon has been reported in 10 to 44 percent of patients with SLE (Dimant et al., 1979; Estes and

Christian, 1971; Fessel, 1974; Harvey et al., 1954; Hochberg et al., 1985; Tuffanelli and Dubois, 1964). It precedes the other manifestations of the disease by several years in a few patients, but it usually develops later in the course of the disease.

Clinical Picture

Criteria for the diagnosis of SLE have been recommended by the American Rheumatism Association (Tan et al., 1982) (Table 6–4). SLE should be considered in a young woman with Raynaud's phenomenon who has a photosensitive malar (butterfly) face rash, arthralgias or arthritis, alopecia, seizures, pleurisy, pericarditis, nephritis, or psychosis. An old adage stated that a young woman with Raynaud's phenomenon and epilepsy should be considered to have SLE until proved otherwise. It has been found that SLE patients who have Raynaud's phenomenon manifest a greater incidence of arthritis, malar rash, and photosensitivity but a lesser degree of renal disease and a better survival rate than patients without Raynaud's phenomenon (Dimant et al., 1979). Avascular necrosis of bone has also been reported to be more frequent in SLE patients with Raynaud's phenomenon (Smith et al., 1976), but this finding has not been confirmed (Dimant et al., 1979).

Laboratory Studies

Anemia is a common, nonspecific finding in the laboratory work-up. Leukopenia occurs in about 50 percent of patients, and thrombocytopenia is not uncommon.

Table 6–4. American Rheumatism Association 1982 Revised Criteria for Classification of Systemic Lupus Erythematosus

For the purpose of identifying patients in clinical studies, a person shall be said to have SLE if any 4 or more of the 11 criteria are present serially or simultaneously, during any interval of observation.

Malar butterfly rash
Discoid rash
Photosensitivity
Oral ulcers
Arthritis (nonerosive)
Serositis (pleuritis or pericarditis)
Renal involvement (persistent proteinuria > 0.5 g/day or cellular casts of any type)
Neurological disorder (seizures, psychosis without other reason)
Hematological disorder
    Hemolytic anemia: with reticulocytosis *or*
    Leukopenia < 4000 cells/μl on two or more occasions *or*
    Lymphopenia < 1500 cells/μl on two or more occasions *or*
    Thrombocytopenia < 100,000/μl in the absence of offending drugs
Immunological disorder
    Positive LE cell preparation *or*
    Anti-DNA: presence of antibody to untreated DNA in abnormal titer *or*
    Anti-Sm: presence of antibody to Sm nuclear antigen *or*
    False-positive serologic test for syphilis known to be positive for at least 6 months and confirmed
      by more specific tests
Antinuclear antibody: an abnormal titer of antinuclear antibody by immunofluorescence or equivalent assay at any point in time and in the absence of drugs known to be associated with "drug-induced lupus" syndrome

Source: Tan et al. (1982).

If a circulating anticoagulant (due to anticardiolipin antibodies) is present, the partial thromboplastin time is prolonged. The ESR is often elevated. Blood cells and red blood cell casts may be found in the urine. Complement levels are often depressed. A large number of antibodies are present that react to cells and their nuclear and cytoplasmic constituents. The antinuclear antibodies are often homogeneous in pattern, and antibodies to double-stranded DNA and Smith (Sm) antigen are characteristic.

Pathology

Pathologically, many of the clinical manifestations are due to vasculitis involving arterioles and venules, although large-artery (coronary, femoral) involvement does occur. Fibrinoid necrosis of blood vessels and an eosinophilic amorphous material is commonly seen in the tissues and blood vessels.

Etiology

The cause of SLE is unknown, but SLE is considered to be an autoimmune disease, with the patient reacting against his or her own tissues. Immune complexes deposited in various organs and tissues produce an inflammatory response. A similar syndrome occurs following use of certain drugs, e.g., procainamide, hydralazine, hydantoins, and isoniazid.

Treatment

In some studies Raynaud's phenomenon has improved after treatment of the SLE with corticosteroids (Kenamore et al., 1968).

Polymyositis/Dermatomyositis

Polymyositis and dermatomyositis, inflammatory diseases of skeletal muscle, are characterized by symmetrical weakness of the proximal muscles. They occur most commonly during the fifth and sixth decades and appear twice as frequently in women as in men. Approximately one-third of patients have Raynaud's phenomenon. In addition to the muscle weakness, there may be dysphagia, dysarthria, arthralgias, arthritis, and an erythematous skin rash. A purplish (heliotrope) discoloration occurs on the upper eyelids and, when present, aids in the diagnosis. Serum levels of creatine phosphokinase and aldolase are often markedly elevated. Muscle biopsy shows fiber degeneration, necrosis, and fibrosis with a mononuclear cell infiltrate. Boylan and Sokoloff (1960) described sclerotic changes in small vessels and arterioles in two children with dermatomyositis. The changes were noted in striated muscle, skin, and the gastrointestinal tract. The authors suggested that these vascular abnormalities were responsible for development of the disease. However, in polymyositis, there is no small vessel necrosis.

Rheumatoid Arthritis and Sjögren's Syndrome

Raynaud's phenomenon may occur in conjunction with rheumatoid arthritis and Sjögren's syndrome. With rheumatoid arthritis, pathology specimens may show obliterative intimal proliferation of the digital arteries (Scott et al., 1961). Vasomotor instability manifested by mottled, cool, sweaty hands on exposure to cold is more common than Raynaud's phenomenon. Focal ischemic lesions and microinfarctions appear as small brown areas in the periungual areas and digital pulp. Arteriograms in these patients with vascular manifestations almost always show occlusions of one or more digital arteries (Laws et al., 1963).

Dry eyes and mouth and enlargement of salivary or lacrimal glands suggest Sjögren's syndrome. Secondary Sjögren's syndrome may occur in association with several diseases but most frequently rheumatoid arthritis and SLE. Patients with primary Sjögren's syndrome, rheumatoid arthritis, and SLE may test positive for rheumatoid factor and antinuclear antibody. However, most patients with primary Sjögren's syndrome possess antibody to SS-A antigen, and about 50 percent of these patients have antibody to SS-B (Fox et al., 1984). These antibodies are seen less frequently in patients with rheumatoid arthritis but are not infrequent in those with SLE when Sjögren's syndrome is also present. Patients with primary Sjögren's syndrome also have a high frequency of histocompatibility antigen HLA-DR3 and lack antibodies to salivary gland ducts, whereas rheumatoid arthritis patients with secondary Sjögren's syndrome have an increased frequency of HLA-DR4 and possess antibodies to salivary ducts. Primary Sjögren's syndrome shows much overlap with SLE in terms of autoantibodies and HLA-DR3, but antibodies to DNA are relatively rare and patients lack sufficient features to meet the criteria for the diagnosis of SLE (Table 6–4).

Mixed Connective Tissue Disease

As the name implies, mixed connective tissue disease (MCTD) has many clinical features in common with SLE, scleroderma, dermatomyositis, and rheumatoid arthritis (Sharp, 1975). Patients often have arthralgias, arthritis, myopathy, and pulmonary or renal involvement. Raynaud's phenomenon may occur in up to 85 percent of patients (Nimelstein et al., 1980; Sharp, 1975) and may precede other manifestations of the disease by several years (Ellman et al., 1981). Swelling of the dorsum of the hands and fingers, producing a tapered or sausage-shaped appearance of the digits, is typical of the disease. Antinuclear antibodies of a speckled pattern are often present, and a high titer of antibodies to ribonuclease-extractable antigens (ENA) usually develops during the course of the disease. Rheumatoid factor and an elevated ESR are also common. Marked improvement in the disease manifestations and Raynaud's phenomenon have been reported with steroid therapy (Ellmann et al., 1981; Sharp, 1975), but not all patients respond (Johansson et al., 1981).

Psoriasis and Raynaud's Phenomenon

Reeves and colleagues (1986) described two patients who presented with both Raynaud's phenomenon and psoriasis. Both patients had serum autoantibodies to U1 and U2 small nuclear ribonucleoproteins. The Raynaud's phenomenon appeared before the psoriasis in only one of the patients. The unique autoantibodies were not found in patients with only psoriasis or Raynaud's phenomenon. The two patients had no other manifestations of a connective tissue disease, but the authors suggested that it may be a new type.

RAYNAUD'S PHENOMENON AND PRIMARY
PULMONARY HYPERTENSION

Several patients have been reported to have pulmonary hypertension and Raynaud's phenomenon with no apparent etiology for either the pulmonary or the peripheral circulatory disease (Celoria et al., 1960; Smith and Kroop, 1957; Winters et al., 1964). This concurrence has led to hypotheses that vasospasm may occur in the pulmonary and digital circulation perhaps owing to a neurohumoral mechanism. Recurrent episodes of vasospasm would then lead to permanent pathological change in the small vessels of the lungs and digits. Pulmonary hypertension is associated with the connective tissue diseases with or without Raynaud's phenomenon.

Pathological changes in the lungs have included marked intimal thickening or concentric proliferation in the arterioles (Celoria et al., 1960; Smith and Kroop, 1957; Winters et al., 1964) and intimal cellular proliferation in vessels less than 300 μm (Celoria et al., 1960). Arteriosclerosis of the larger pulmonary arteries has also been present in some patients. Skin or muscle biopsies have shown no pathological changes.

Pulmonary function studies in patients with Raynaud's phenomenon have been variable. Wise and co-workers (1982) found an increase in carbon monoxide diffusing capacity during whole-body cooling in patients with primary Raynaud's disease and Raynaud's phenomenon with SLE but not in those with scleroderma. If reflex pulmonary vasoconstriction occurred the diffusing capacity would not increase, whereas it would if accentuated peripheral vasoconstriction shifted blood volume from the systemic to the pulmonary vasculature. Miller (1983) also found an 8 percent increase in the diffusing capacity in patients with primary Raynaud's disease during ice water immersion of one hand but no change in normal subjects or patients with scleroderma. Shuck and co-workers (1985) concluded that pulmonary vasospasm with transient pulmonary hypertension did not occur in patients with scleroderma and Raynaud's phenomenon, as no significant change in mean pulmonary artery pressure or pulmonary vascular resistance was found during immersion of a hand in cold water. Contrary to the above studies, Fahey and colleagues (1984) reported that patients with primary Raynaud's disease had a decrease in carbon monoxide diffusing capacity with immersion of one hand in 15°C water. They found that patients with secondary Raynaud's phenomenon had a decreased diffusing capacity with no stimulation but no change with the cold test. Thus the issue of increased pulmonary vascular sensitivity to cold in patients with primary Raynaud's disease is still unsettled.

The question remains if in some patients primary pulmonary hypertension and digital vasospasm are connected by a common mechanism that induces vasoconstriction. Walcott and colleagues (1970) found that 30 percent of their patients with primary pulmonary hypertension had Raynaud's phenomenon, as did 10 percent of 82 women reported by Fuster et al. (1984). The latter figure (10 percent) is no different from the occurrence of primary Raynaud's disease in the general population (see Chap. 2). Fisher and co-workers (1987), while studying the effect of nifedipine in 24 patients with primary and secondary pulmonary hypertension, found that the six patients with Raynaud's phenomenon had the most significant decrease in resting mean pulmonary artery pressure and pulmonary vascular resistance. They postulated that it could be due to reversible pulmonary vasoconstriction, although prior chronic vasodilator therapy may have preserved pulmonary vasoreactivity. It can be concluded therefore that the evidence is not strong enough to state that a separate disease entity exists that manifests only pulmonary and digital vasospasm.

TRAUMATIC VASOSPASTIC DISEASE

Raynaud's phenomenon caused by use of vibratory tools or constant repetitive trauma to the digits has been termed Raynaud's phenomenon of occupational origin, traumatic vasospastic disease, or vibration-induced white fingers. It has been reported in workers who use pneumatic hammers, chain saws, chisels, riveting machines, road drills, pounding and lasting machines, brush saws, and sewing machines (Reiss, 1969). It may also occur in telephone operators, typists, pianists, and meat cutters. It is probably the commonest cause of Raynaud's phenomenon in men.

Incidence and Predisposing Factors

A large proportion of workers with vibratory tools develop vasospastic symptoms. Various studies have reported an incidence of 30 to 84 percent of workers (Chatterjee et al., 1978; Futatsuka et al., 1985a; Hellstrom and Andersen, 1972; Olsen and Nielsen, 1979; Theriault et al., 1982). In these same studies, Raynaud's phenomenon occurred in 2.3 to 14.0 percent of workers who did not use vibratory tools; the highest incidence occurred in outdoor workers (Hellstrom and Andersen, 1972). The mean time of onset after use of vibratory tools averaged 6.4 to 8.0 years, with a range of 1 to 19 years; Futatsuka and Ueno (1985) calculated that most patients had 6000 to 7000 hours of exposure. Theriault and co-workers (1982) reported a greater risk for smokers. Almost half of the workers who filet ice-frozen fish and frequently rewarm their fingers develop Raynaud's phenomenon within 2 to 3 years compared to only 12 percent of workers chronically exposed to cold (Mackiewicz and Piskorz, 1977). It was blamed on exposure to great differences of temperature, but the hands may also be exposed to constant trauma in this occupation. A family history of Raynaud's phenomenon, previous injuries to the arm, and a cold climate also have been predisposing factors.

Clinical Picture

The vasospastic episodes involve blanching and numbness of the fingers; pain and cyanosis are said to be uncommon (Gurdjian and Walker, 1945; Hellstrom and Andersen, 1972). The hand exposed to the tool is usually more severely involved, although the opposite hand has been described as being more extensively affected among some workers (Olsen and Nielsen, 1979). The involvement of the hands is often not symmetrical. The feet are not involved. Attacks are produced by both use of the vibratory tools and exposure to cold. Emotional stimuli have not been implicated. Hyvarinen and colleagues (1973) reported digital vasoconstriction in lumberjacks with the disease when they were exposed to chain-saw noise. The syndrome does not progress to gangrene or loss of fingers; workers often continue in the occupation for years despite the vasospastic attacks. Hashimoto and Craig (1980) have reported one case of acrosclerosis with digital ulcers.

Associated Clinical Syndromes

Some authorities consider the Raynaud's phenomenon of traumatic vasospastic disease to be part of a syndrome involving the nerves, muscles, and joints, as patients often complain of elbow and shoulder pains or weakness (Ashe et al., 1962; Futatsuka et al., 1985a; Marshall et al., 1954). Banister and Smith (1972) found a significant loss in manipulative skills in their patients, but Hellstrom and Andersen (1972) could find no evidence of injury to peripheral nerves, muscles, bones, or joints by tactile two-point discrimination, maximal isometric muscle strength, or radiography. Hearing loss has been reported by Iki and co-workers (1983, 1987) and Matoba and colleagues (1977). Miyakita and co-workers (1987) showed that noise may play a part in inducing digital vasoconstriction along with local exposure to vibration, and that hand vibration may affect hearing thresholds. Several investigators consider that the central nervous system is involved and have reported a high incidence of headache, palmar hyperhidrosis, forgetfulness, fatigability, tinnitus, impotence, dizziness, and other symptoms (Futatsuka et al., 1985a; Matoba et al., 1977). Matoba and co-workers (1977) also reported electroencephalographic abnormalities in 18 percent of their patients.

Pathology

Pathology studies are few. Gurdjian and Walker (1945) reported that biopsies of the fingers were normal in five patients. Ashe and co-workers (1962) described medial muscular hypertrophy and moderate to marked subintimal fibrosis of the digital vessels. Angiography revealed tapered arteries in the forearms of their patients. Takeuchi and Imanishi (1984) also reported thickening of the muscular layer of the arteries and hypertrophy of muscle cells but without fibrosis of the intima. Matoba and co-workers (1977) described the nailfold capillaries, examined microscopically, as being smaller and more tortuous than in normal subjects. Okada and associates (1987) exposed rat hind limbs to local vibration of 60 Hz for 4 hours a day for 30 or 90 days. In the animals exposed for 90 days, there was disruption of the internal elastic lamina in small arteries and focal cell proliferation, with regenerative formation of collagen and elastic fibers. Thickening of the intima led to obstruction of the lumen, and proliferation of arterial smooth muscle cells and numerous collagen and elastic fibers were seen by electron microscopy. No changes were apparent at 30 days. Whole blood viscosity was also significantly increased in the rats at 90 days.

Pathophysiology

How the use of vibratory tools induces vasospastic attacks is not known. Futatsuka and Ueno (1985) considered that the frequency, level, direction, and duration of the vibration as well as the grip and the environmental temperature are important. It is true that several studies correlate the duration of vibration exposure with the incidence of the syndrome, and that the severity of the syndrome increases with hand-tool operating time (Miyashita et al., 1983). In dogs and rats, Azuma and co-workers (1978) showed that the dose-response relation of excised femoral arteries to norepinephrine was enhanced after acute vibratory stimulation; the enhancement depended on the frequency amplitude and the duration of the stimulation. The same workers (Azuma et al., 1980) showed that a vibratory stimulus first reduced the peripheral resistance and the response to norepinephrine in the dog hindlimb but that enhancement occurred 1 hour after stimulation. Whereas Ryan and Salter (1977) reported an increase in hand blood flow with a vibratory stimulus of 80 Hz, Welsh (1980) found a decrease in digital blood flow with 40 to 200 Hz that was greatest at 125 Hz. Only the finger being vibrated showed this reaction. Farkkila and Pyykko (1979) found vasoconstriction in fingers of patients with traumatic vasospastic disease at 60 to 200 Hz that correlated with the severity of the disease. Olsen and Petring (1988) reported that men with this disease and normal controls showed a similar vasoconstriction response in the digits (Xe^{133} disappearance rate) to 125 Hz which was abolished by proximal nerve blockade. A central sympathetic vasoconstrictor reflex elicited by vibration was therefore indicated. Hyvarinen and co-workers (1973) pointed out that the dominant frequency of chain saws is 125 Hz, which falls in the region where the pacinian corpuscles are especially sensitive to vibration. They postulated that chronic overexcitation of these corpuscles may produce the vasospastic reactions through a reflex linkage with the sympathetic nervous system. Because similar reactions occur in the hand not exposed to vibration, the linkage may be in the central nervous system. Stewart and Goda (1970) postulated that the syndrome was due to deposition of callus on the palmar surfaces of the fingers, causing a decrease in blood volume in the capillaries, which in turn would increase the susceptibility to vasospasm on vibratory or cold stimulation. However, other workers who develop calluses on their fingers not using vibratory tools do not develop the syndrome.

Okada and co-workers (1983) found a large increase in plasma cyclic guanosine 3',5'-monophosphate in patients with vibration disease during a cold pressor test; it did not occur in normals, and it was suppressed by phentolamine or atropine. They postulated that cholinergic or α-adrenergic receptor responses are enhanced. Stimulation of α_1-adrenoceptors by phenylephrine was found to be depressed in the digits of patients compared to control subjects, whereas the response to α_2-adrenoceptor activation was intact, leading to the possibility that vibration may damage some receptor types (Ekenvall and Lindblad, 1986b). Futatsuka and co-workers (1983) reported that finger blood flow in patients was the same as in controls during body heating; because the calculated peripheral resistance of the fingers was not different during reflex vasoconstriction, they considered that there was no evidence that excess responses to cold were secondary to hypertrophy of the vessel walls. However, a true measure of digital peripheral resistance is difficult to determine. A variety of platelet aggregation studies were reported as normal in 13 subjects in the early stages of the disease (Bovenzi, 1986). As with primary Raynaud's disease, cold-induced vasodilation is still present (Hellstrom et al., 1970). It may be concluded that no final answer is available; as with primary Raynaud's disease, there is the possibility of abnormal α- or β-adrenoceptor activity, hyperactivity of the sympathetic nervous system, hypertrophy of the digital vessels, or an abnormal response of the vascular smooth muscle to normal vasoconstrictor or vibratory stimuli.

Diagnostic Tests

Several investigators have presented evidence that these patients have an increased responsiveness to normal vasoconstrictor stimuli. Many tests for diagnosis have been used, but no test has a high sensitivity and specificity. Abnormally low digital systolic blood pressure, finger temperature, and finger blood flow in response to ischemic cooling as well as the rewarming time after cooling have been demonstrated in these patients as in patients with other types of Raynaud's phenomenon (Juul and Nielsen, 1981; Olsen et al., 1985). The digital rewarming test after cooling and after 10°C water immersion plus ischemia have been shown to have good group reproducibility in normal subjects and patients (Hack et al., 1986). However, the tests were not useful for diagnosis in individual cases. Olsen and co-workers (1982, 1985) also found this hyperresponsiveness in patients' fingers without symptoms and that a sympathetic block of the finger returned the response to normal. Juul and Nielsen (1981) described the hyperresponsiveness as being greater than in patients with primary Raynaud's disease. Ekenvall and Lindblad (1986a) found a diagnostic sensitivity of only 74 to 79 percent using the finger systolic pressure measurement during body and local finger cooling in 111 patients. Olsen (1988), using similar tests plus an evaluation of finger color after an ischemic cold stimulus, reported similar levels of sensitivity and specificity.

Prognosis

The prognosis for abatement of this disease is variable. Although some improvement may occur after use of the tools has ceased, the hands usually remain sensitive to cold exposure (Ashe et al., 1962; Ekenvall and Carlson, 1987; Gurdjian and Walker, 1945). Futatsuka and co-workers (1985b) found that 50.2 percent of chainsaw workers still had the syndrome 12 years after cessation of tool use. The same group (Futatsuka and Ueno, 1985) studied Japanese forestry workers and found that 13.5 percent recovered while still exposed to chain saws, 12.2 percent recovered within 1 year of cessation of tool use, and 74.3 percent still had the syndrome 2 years after cessation. In contrast, 59 percent of brush-saw workers, who work during a warmer season than chain-saw users, fully recovered within 5 years and 71 percent in 10 years (Futatsuka, 1984); in another study, symptoms improved or disappeared in forestry workers if exposure to vibration was reduced or stopped over a 5-year period (Olsen and Nielsen, 1988).

Treatment and Prophylaxis

Recommendations for prevention and treatment of the syndrome include meticulous training in the easiest ways to use the tools, use of multiple layers of warm gloves inside an outer waterproof glove, and frequent changing of gloves if the hands become wet (Ashe et al., 1962). Workers should also wear warm clothing. The incidence of the disease has decreased with the introduction of antivibratory saws and limiting the duration of tool use to 2 hours per day (Futatsuka and Ueno, 1985). Drug therapy has not been extensively studied. Diltiazem 30 mg three times a day significantly decreased a variety of subjective symptoms and improved the rewarming time of hands immersed in 10°C water in an open trial of 17 patients with vibration disease (Matoba et al., 1982).

CARPAL TUNNEL SYNDROME

Patients with carpal tunnel syndrome may present with Raynaud's phenomenon or acrocyanosis (Linscheid et al., 1967). The phenomenon may precede other manifestations of the carpal tunnel syndrome by 6 to 12 months (Serra et al., 1985). Vasospastic attacks may be mild to severe; only the first three fingers may be involved. In severe cases the feet and nose may also be involved, indicating an underlying disease that is also affecting the carpal tunnel. Rare instances of persistent discoloration of the fingers with bullae formation and small areas of necrosis may occur (Aratari et al., 1984). No underlying cause for Raynaud's phenomenon except the carpal tunnel syndrome is found in almost 50 percent of patients. Other nerve entrapment syndromes, e.g., ulnar nerve entrapment at the elbow, may also induce vasospastic attacks.

Etiology, Anatomy, Pathophysiology

There are many causes of the carpal tunnel syndrome (Table 6–5). In a large number of patients, no underlying reason for the syndrome can be found. The carpal tunnel is formed by the carpal bones and is covered by the transverse carpal ligament running across the anterior aspect of the wrist (Fig. 6–5). It contains the median nerve and artery and three muscle tendons in bursae. Any increase in pres-

Table 6–5. Causes of Carpal Tunnel Syndrome

Idiopathic (no cause found)	Infections
Systemic diseases	Infections of forearm or hand
Acromegaly	Tuberculosis
Myxedema	Histoplasmosis
Diabetes mellitus	Miscellaneous
Amyloidosis	Pregnancy
Gout	Median artery thrombosis
Rheumatoid arthritis	Hemorrhage into tunnel
Osteoarthritis	Fractures or dislocations
Dermatomyositis	Bee sting
Scleroderma	Nonspecific tenosynovitis
Lupus erythematosus	Anomalous or accessory muscles
Sarcoidosis	Hemodialysis (?amyloid)
Tumors	
Neuromas	
Ganglions	
Fibromas	
Lipomas	

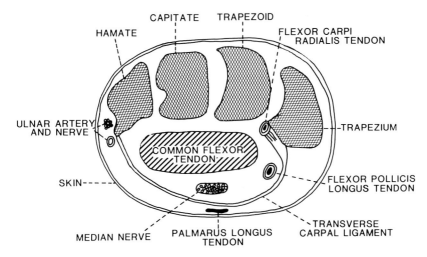

Fig. 6-5. Transverse section at the wrist illustrating the structure and contents of the carpal canal. The median nerve lies in a tight space bounded by the transverse carpal ligament and the muscle tendon sheaths.

sure within this tight compartment can damage the median nerve. Gelberman and co-workers (1981) found the intracarpal canal pressures greatly increased in patients with carpal tunnel syndrome compared to control subjects. With most etiologies there is swelling, inflammation, or deposition or infiltration of tissue in the tunnel leading to compression of the median nerve. Amyloid deposition has been found in hemodialysis patients (Walts et al., 1985). Dekel and colleagues (1980), using computed tomography, found that women had smaller carpal canals than men and the symptomatic patients had even narrower canals than women, especially proximally. This finding may be one explanation for the greater incidence in women than men. It may be an inherited problem, as there was no correlation of canal size with age. Bleecker and co-workers (1985) found that carpal canal size was smaller in electricians who developed the syndrome than in normal subjects.

Clinical Picture

Patients complain of numbness, burning, or tingling in the thumb, index, and middle fingers. The symptoms are usually most annoying at night and often awaken the patient. It is common for pain to radiate to the arm or shoulder, creating confusion with the thoracic outlet syndrome. Most often symptoms are bilateral, but the right hand is more often affected than the left when the disorder is unilateral.

Physical Examination

Examination may reveal weakness and atrophy of the thenar eminence, as the innervation of the abductor pollicis brevis and opponens pollicis muscles is involved. When sensory changes are present, they are only distal to the wrist. Anhidrosis of fingers may occur.

Diagnosis

The diagnosis is made by nerve conduction studies, which reveal prolongation of median nerve sensory latencies and decreased sensory potentials, which occur in 85 to 95 percent of patients (Hoffman, 1975; Stevens, 1987). Delayed motor latencies at the wrist occur in about two-thirds of patients. Tinel's sign (which is the reproduction of symptoms in the innervated fingers induced by tapping the median nerve at the wrist) or Phalen's sign (which produces symptoms by maximal wrist flexion for 1 minute) are often positive but have low sensitivity and specificity (Heller et al., 1986). However, reproduction of symptoms by flexion or extension of the wrist is sometimes helpful in the diagnosis.

Treatment

Various treatments have been advocated for correction of this syndrome. Relief by injecting 25 to 50 mg of hydrocortisone in 1 ml into the carpal tunnel has been used as treatment as well as for diagnosis (Hamlin and Lehman, 1967). In one prospective study, a single injection of 30 mg of triamcinolone and splinting the wrist for 3 weeks resulted in cure of 22 percent of 50 hands (Gelberman et al., 1980). In another study, 28 percent of 492 hands were completely relieved of symptoms by corticosteroid injections (Stevens, 1987). The patients with good results usually had mild symptoms for less than 1 year, normal sensation, normal thenar muscle mass and strength, and only a 1- to 2-msec prolongation of nerve conduction velocity. Immobilization of the wrist in a cast or splint has been advocated and has produced variable results. Diuretics may be of value during pregnancy, and estrogens have been used in postmenopausal women (Layton, 1958). Vitamin B_6 has been recommended by Ellis and co-workers (1977), who reported improvement of patients with pyroxidine 100 mg three times a day; they implicated a vitamin B_6 deficiency manifested by decreased erythrocyte glutamic oxaloacetic transaminase. However, Smith and colleagues (1984) found normal pyridoxal and pyridoxal phosphate by plasma and neutrophil assays in their patients. Four of their six patients claimed partial symptomatic relief, but there was no consistent improvement in clinical findings or neurophysiological measurements on 100 mg of pyridoxine daily. Surgical decompression of the carpal tunnel by section of the transverse ligament remains the preferred treatment, with most studies reporting an 80 to 90 percent cure rate (Taylor, 1971). However, in patients who have Raynaud's phenomenon, the vasospastic attacks may or may not be helped (Linscheid et al., 1967; Serra et al., 1985).

THORACIC OUTLET SYNDROME

Raynaud's phenomenon can be a major manifestation of neurovascular compression in the thoracic outlet. In one series (McGough et al., 1979), 5.3 percent of 1200 patients with different types of the thoracic outlet syndrome had vasospastic attacks. Beyer and Wright (1951) reported that 20 of 52 patients with the hyperabduction syndrome had Raynaud's phenomenon. Fingertip ulcers may also occur in these syndromes.

Anatomy

The subclavian artery in the neck passes over the first rib behind the scalenus anticus muscle and in front of the scalenus medius muscle. It then courses under the subclavius muscle and clavicle into the axilla underneath the pectoralis minor muscle. The subclavian vein accompanies the artery but lies anterior to the scalenus anticus muscle. The brachial plexus runs posterolateral to the vessels. Therefore the neurovascular bundle can be compressed by an extra cervical rib, by the scalenus muscles (scalenus anticus syndrome), between the first thoracic rib and clavicle (costoclavicular syndrome), or by the pectoralis minor muscle tendon (hyperabduction syndrome). Congenital abnormalities of the thoracic outlet structures, fibrous bands, and variations of insertion of the scalenus muscles contribute to or are the cause of the disorder in some patients.

Cervical Ribs

Cervical ribs occur in 0.5 to 1.0 percent of the population, but only about 10 percent cause symptoms (Adson and Coffey, 1927). These cervical ribs may vary in length and width, and they may be bony or fibrous. Because of this extra rib, the subclavian artery passes higher than usual as it emerges from the thorax, making it susceptible to distortion or kinking. Direct compression of the artery by the rib or even compression of sympathetic fibers in the brachial plexus could be the cause of Raynaud's phenomenon (Telford and Mottershead, 1948). Subclavian artery thrombosis or postcompression dilation may occur with embolism to the distal extremity (Banis et al., 1977).

Scalenus Anticus Syndrome

A fibrous band at the border of the scalenus anticus muscle is common, but anatomic variations in its insertion may compress the subclavian artery or brachial plexus. Infrequently, the artery may pass through the belly of the muscle and be directly compressed during muscle contraction. The subclavian vein is not affected in this syndrome or with cervical ribs because it passes anterior to the muscle.

Costoclavicular Syndrome

Congenital or acquired abnormalities of the first thoracic rib or clavicle may cause this syndrome, but often no abnormalities are found. The neurovascular bundle is compressed between the clavicle and first rib in certain positions, especially when the shoulders are pulled back or down. Subclavian arterial or venous thrombosis may occur.

Hyperabduction Syndrome

Although no abnormalities of the thoracic outlet are present, compression of the neurovascular bundle by the pectoralis minor tendon is probably the cause (Lord and Rosati, 1958). Axillary venous thrombosis may occur.

Pathophysiology

Raynaud's phenomenon has been considered to be due to vasospasm in the digits caused by irritation of the sympathetic nerves in the neurovascular bundle in the thoracic outlet. However, some investigators believe that it represents thromboemboli in the digital arteries from the subclavian artery. Swinton and co-workers (1970) found subclavian artery thrombi in three patients with unilateral Raynaud's phenomenon who had a cervical–first rib anomaly. There are no pathology studies in a large group of patients to support this contention, and Raynaud's phenomenon is often bilateral.

Symptoms and Signs

Neurological symptoms are much more frequent than vascular symptoms in these syndromes, although the incidence of vascular problems in the hyperabduction syndrome is high (Beyer and Wright, 1951). Pain, numbness, and paresthesias of the neck, arm, or hand are common. Discoloration and swelling of the arm or hand may result from subclavian vein compression. Digital ulcers are sometimes present. The inner arm and fourth and fifth fingers are often the most symptomatic owing to compression of nerves C8 and T1. When Raynaud's phenomenon is present, the manifestations are typical, and vasospastic attacks are precipitated by cold and emotions.

Although cervical ribs or other congenital abnormalities may be present from birth, symptoms in all these syndromes usually develop in the age group 20 to 40 years of age. This pattern is considered secondary to the drooping of the shoulder girdle with age and sometimes, in women, to heavy breasts. Patients often notice that symptoms are aggravated by certain positions of the arms. Painters and mechanics have symptoms when they have to work above their heads; women have more symptoms when combing their hair. Patients with the hyperabduction syndrome often awake at night with numb, weak arms or hands.

Physical findings include systolic bruits in the supraclavicular or infraclavicular fossae either in the neutral position or with the maneuvers described below. Supraclavicular or axillary area tenderness has been present in up to 93 percent of patients (McGough et al., 1979). Weakness of hand grip, triceps muscle, or interosseous hand muscles may be present (Roos, 1982). Hypesthesia to touch and pinprick on the inner forearm and ulnar side of the hand and fingers also occurs. Arterial pulses in the arms are usually present and normal.

Diagnosis

The diagnosis of the thoracic outlet syndromes is often difficult, with some experts recommending reliance on the history and physical examination; others consider nerve conduction studies important as well. There are three maneuvers that should be performed on patients suspected of having a thoracic outlet syndrome. It is important that symptoms or signs (paleness and numbness of the hand) be reproduced by these maneuvers; loss of the radial pulse occurs in many normal subjects (Conn, 1974; Wright, 1945).

Adson's maneuver (Adson, 1947) involves having the patient sit in a comfortable position (Fig. 6–6). With the neck extended fully and the chin turned toward the side being examined, a deep breath is taken. A positive test includes production of symptoms or a pale hand; the radial pulse should be lost or diminished. It is valuable to repeat the test with the head turned to the opposite side. Adson's maneuver may be positive with cervical ribs or the scalenus anticus syndrome.

With the hyperabduction maneuver, the radial pulse is continuously palpated with the patient sitting (Fig. 6–7). The arm is then slowly hyperabducted; i.e., it is raised above head level and rotated slightly away from the body. Reproduction of symptoms or pallor of the hand constitute a positive test; the radial pulse should be obliterated or diminished. A systolic bruit may also be produced in the supra- or infraclavicular area or over the axillary artery during the maneuver.

The costoclavicular maneuver is performed with the patient sitting (Fig. 6–8). The patient is requested to pull the shoulders backward and downward into an exaggerated military position. It is also helpful to have the patient hold a deep breath. Production of symptoms or pallor of the hand indicate an abnormal test; the radial pulse is diminished or obliterated.

Roos (1982) used a test in which the patient exercised his hands for 3 minutes with the elbow at right angles to the thorax and the forearms flexed at a 90-degree angle. Roos found this test diagnostic for all thoracic outlet syndromes.

The presence of cervical ribs or other bony abnormalities may be proved by radiographs of the chest and cervical spine. Apical lesions of the lung, which can cause similar symptoms, can also be ruled out by a chest film.

Fig. 6–6. Demonstration of Adson's maneuver in a normal subject. The neck is fully extended with the head turned toward the side being examined. The subject takes a deep breath while the examiner palpates the radial artery, observes the color of the hand, and notes any symptoms.

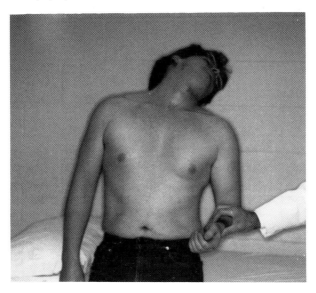

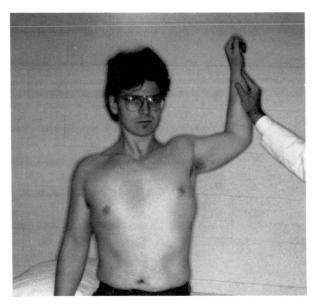

Fig. 6–7. Demonstration of the hyperabduction maneuver in a normal subject. The radial pulse is continuously palpated by the examiner while the arm is slowly raised above head level and rotated slightly away from the body. The color of the hand is observed and any symptoms noted.

Fig. 6–8. Demonstration of the costoclavicular maneuver in a normal subject. The shoulders are pulled backward and downward in an exaggerated military position, and the subject is requested to hold a deep breath. The examiner continually palpates the radial artery, observes the color of the hands, and notes any symptoms.

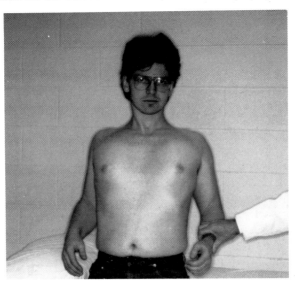

Nerve conduction studies yield variable results but do help to rule out the carpal tunnel syndrome. McGough and co-workers (1979) reported slowing of ulnar nerve conduction velocity across the thoracic outlet in 61 percent of 1200 patients. Urschel and Razzuk (1972) considered this test abnormal in most patients and based therapeutic decisions on the degree of abnormality. Somatosensory evoked potentials of the median and ulnar nerves in the neutral and stressed positions were abnormal in 74 percent of 80 patients and correlated with postoperative improvement in the study of Machleder and co-workers (1987). Some experts do not consider nerve conduction studies and electromyography to be of value when diagnosing the disease or choosing patients for surgical treatment (Roos, 1987).

Arteriography or venography is useful only if vascular occlusions or postcompression aneurysms with emboli are suspected.

Treatment

Treatment of the thoracic outlet syndrome has cured or alleviated some patients who had the manifestations of Raynaud's phenomenon (Beyer and Wright, 1951; McGough et al., 1979). Most authorities agree that conservative therapy should be tried first, as up to 70 percent of patients do improve (Rosati and Lord, 1961; Urschel et al., 1968). Positions should be avoided that aggravate the symptoms. Exercises to strengthen the muscles of the shoulder girdle and improve posture often yield remarkably good results. They help relieve the compression on the neurovascular bundle. Sleeping posture is also important for maintaining the shoulder girdle in an abducted and slightly elevated position (McGough, 1979). In the hyperabduction syndrome, the arms may have to be restrained in bed to keep them away from a hyperabducted position during sleep. Surgical treatment consists in removal of the first rib (or cervical rib) with or without division of the scalenus anticus muscle; various approaches have been used. If patients are carefully selected and have failed conservative therapy, 80 percent (McGough et al., 1979) to 95 percent (Roos, 1982; Urschel and Razzuk, 1972) of patients have good to excellent results. Patients with significant vascular symptoms and those with cervical ribs are said to have excellent relief of symptoms with surgery (Conn, 1974).

HYPOTHENAR HAMMER SYNDROME (ULNAR ARTERY THROMBOSIS)

Ulnar artery occlusion due to trauma should always be considered in patients who present with Raynaud's phenomenon, especially when only one hand is afflicted. About 2 cm distal to the wrist, the ulnar artery is vulnerable to acute and chronic trauma, as it is protected only by skin, subcutaneous tissue, and the palmar brevis muscle. Patients usually develop this syndrome by hammering with the palms of their hands, but it may also occur after falling, using bowling balls or walkers, or practicing karate (Little and Ferguson, 1972; Millender et al., 1972; Vayssairat et al., 1984). Symptoms may be bilateral owing to ulnar artery occlusions in both hands (Conn et al., 1970).

Incidence

Little and Ferguson (1972) examined 127 mechanics and discovered that 79 admitted to using the palms of the hands for hammering. A positive Allen test confirmed by doppler flow examination was found in 14 percent of the 79. These 11 workers all had symptoms consistent with Raynaud's phenomenon. Mechanics with the syndrome were older and had worked longer at their jobs than the other workers. Of 966 patients evaluated for Raynaud's phenomenon, Vayssairat and co-workers (1987) diagnosed hypothenar hammer syndrome in 1.7 percent.

Pathology

Pathologically, the patient has an occluded, often aneurysmal, ulnar or sometimes radial artery. In some patients the occlusion is in the superficial volar arch, or the whole arch may be occluded. The internal elastic membrane is absent, fragmented, or duplicated. Granulation tissue and localized hemorrhage may extend into the media (Millender et al., 1972). An inflammatory infiltrate of histiocytes, lymphocytes, and fibroblasts may be present in the whole arterial wall (Pineda et al., 1985).

Sex and Age

There is a strong male predominance of this entity. Men in their third to fifth decade of life are usually afflicted, and it is mainly the right hand that is involved.

Clinical Picture

Patients present with Raynaud's phenomenon of one hand, with color changes (pallor or cyanosis) and numbness occurring on exposure to cold. Reactive hyperemia following attacks has not been described. All fingers except the thumbs may be involved; the most affected fingers are the third, fourth, and fifth. There is often a history of chronic or acute trauma to the heel of the hand or of the use of meat cutters, although the inciting trauma may not seem serious to the patient. Occasionally, the patient complains of a tender mass over the hypothenar aspect of the hand. Calluses may be present over the hypothenar eminences, a clue that the hands have been used for hammering. Digital ulcers and gangrene have occurred in some patients. Allen's test is usually positive, but the ulnar and radial arteries palpate normally at the wrist. Doppler flow examination may reveal diminished or absent arterial sounds over the superficial volar arch.

Diagnosis

Angiography, necessary for making the diagnosis, usually reveals irregularity or thrombosis of the ulnar artery in the region of the hamate bone, although more distal occlusions of the arch and multiple digital artery occlusions may be present (Conn et al., 1970; Vayssairat et al., 1984, 1987) (Fig. 6–9). Aneurysms of the ulnar artery or arch have been found in some patients. It has been postulated that the digital artery occlusions are emboli from a thrombus at the site of the proximal trauma.

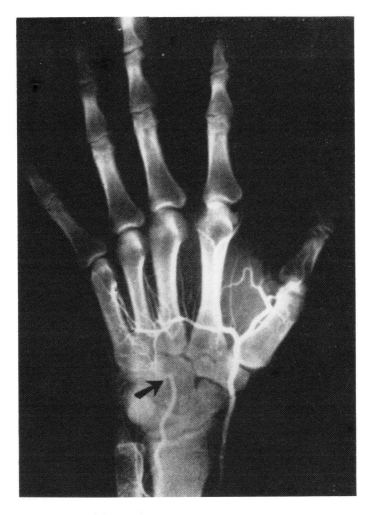

Fig. 6–9. Arteriogram of the right hand of a 38-year-old patient who stacked lumber with the palm of his hand. The arrow points to an occlusion of the distal ulnar artery. This picture is typical of the hypothenar hammer syndrome. *Source:* Conn et al., 1970. Reprinted by permission of the C. V. Mosby Company.

Treatment

Various treatments have been advocated for the hypothenar hammer syndrome. If symptoms are mild, it is best to observe the patient for a few months, as improvement may occur spontaneously probably owing to development of a collateral blood supply (Herndon et al., 1975; Vayssairat et al., 1987). Simple excision of the occluded or aneurysmal portion of the ulnar artery may result in a dramatic cure (Herndon et al., 1975; Millender et al., 1972). Why resection of the diseased segment of vessel is so successful is unknown, but it would cause a local sympathectomy in addition to removing a source for embolization. Stellate ganglion blocks, oral adrenergic blocking agents, or dorsal sympathectomies may also be curative

(Benedict et al., 1974; Conn et al., 1970). Thrombectomy or resection and reanastomosis with or without a graft has been advocated, but reocclusion is common (Benedict et al., 1974; Kleinert and Volianitis, 1965; Millender et al., 1972). Intraarterial fibrinolytic agents have been used with some success for lysing digital artery emboli (Mori et al., 1983; Pineda et al., 1985).

OBSTRUCTIVE ARTERIAL DISEASE

Arteriosclerosis Obliterans

Raynaud's phenomenon may be seen in patients with stenoses or obstructions of large arteries due to arteriosclerosis obliterans. Hines and Barker (1940) mentioned that vasospastic color changes occasionally accompanied the bouts of pain due to ischemic neuritis in patients with this disease. In our experience, vasospastic attacks in patients with arteriosclerosis obliterans are not common, nor is ischemic neuritis a usual accompaniment. Usually only one or two digits of the affected extremity are involved. Attacks of pallor or cyanosis without a red reactive hyperemic phase occur on exposure to cold. Numbness is a common feature. The diagnosis is based on the appearance of vasospastic attacks only in the lower extremity and usually only one limb, the older age of the patient, a history of intermittent claudication, and the absence of pulses in the extremity. It is a common mistake to attribute the appearance of Raynaud's phenomenon involving the fingers in elderly patients to arteriosclerosis obliterans even though normal pulses are present. In these patients, another etiology often becomes apparent. Surgical correction of the obstructive arterial lesion causes the syndrome to disappear.

Thrombangiitis Obliterans

"Vasomotor disturbances suggesting Raynaud's disease" may occur in thromboangiitis obliterans (Allen and Brown, 1928). Allen and Brown observed this syndrome as an early symptom in 2 percent of their 200 patients but found that it may occur in as many as 30 percent of patients during the course of the disease. However, Goodman and colleagues (1965) reported a 57 percent incidence of Raynaud's phenomenon among 80 patients with this disease. Thromboangiitis obliterans (Buerger's disease) is now considered a syndrome that affects medium and small arteries and veins. It has several etiologies, which are unclear, although infections, autoimmune phenomena, and chemical toxicity have been implicated. Young men, 25 to 45 years of age, are affected; it occurs rarely in women. Almost all patients smoke tobacco products, but studies have failed to implicate nicotine as the etiological agent. The lower extremities are affected most commonly, although upper extremities are involved in more than 70 percent of patients. The upper extremity lesions are often asymptomatic (Hirai and Shionoya, 1979); the digital arteries have lesions more frequently than the ulnar or radial arteries. Pathologically, there is inflammation of the walls of the arteries and veins with secondary thromboses. The thrombi may contain foci of leukocytes and surrounding giant cells. In the chronic stage the blood vessels and surrounding tissues become fibrosed.

When a young man who smokes tobacco presents with Raynaud's phenomenon, thromboangiitis obliterans should be considered. If there have been episodes of superficial thrombophlebitis, which occur in about 40 percent of patients, or if intermittent claudication is present, the diagnosis is more likely. Digital ulcers and gangrene are also common. The pain in this disease is often excruciating. On examination, a helpful clue is the absence of pulses at the wrist or ankle. The ulnar artery pulse is often the first vessel missing. Arteriography is characteristic, showing segmental involvement of medium and small arteries with intervening normal areas, an absence of atheroma, and a tree-root pattern of collateral vessels springing from the thrombosed ends of arteries. A definitive diagnosis can be made only by blood vessel biopsy during the acute stages; the chronic stages cannot be distinguished from other diseases ending in perivascular and vascular fibrosis.

Because primary Raynaud's disease is not frequent in men, affects upper extremities more severely, and does not obliterate arterial pulsation at the wrist or ankle, it should not be confused with Raynaud's phenomenon due to thromboangiitis obliterans.

Arterial Emboli

Raynaud's phenomenon may occur in the fingers or toes in a limb that has been involved with arterial emboli in the past. We have seen single digits afflicted with small emboli develop vasospastic attacks after exposure to cold for several years. Resolution of symptoms may correlate with the formation of collateral vessels.

REFLEX SYMPATHETIC DYSTROPHY

Reflex sympathetic dystrophy (RSD) is a syndrome that follows major trauma, e.g., fractures, compression injuries, or surgery, or even the minor trauma of sprains or bruises. In these patients extreme, constant pain persists long after the healing phase. There are signs of disturbed sympathetic activity in the affected extremity. The etiology is unknown, but it may be due to injured sensory fibers transmitting constant signals to the spinal cord, with stimulation of sympathetic centers resulting in decreased and then increased sympathetic outflow to the limb (Drucker et al., 1959). This theory is supported by the fact that sympathectomy performed early in the course of RSD may result in a cure.

There are often two phases of the syndrome. Initially, the painful limb is dry, swollen, and warm. This phase is followed by a vasoconstrictor prolonged stage with a persistently cold, hyperhidrotic, swollen, pale, or even cyanotic extremity. Part or all of a hand or foot or extremity may be involved. During the vasoconstrictor phase there is abnormal sensitivity to cold exposure, and Raynaud's phenomenon may occur. In our experience, actual episodic vasospastic attacks are infrequent. Later in the course, osteoporosis of the bony structures of the involved area (Sudeck's atrophy) may occur.

This syndrome is disabling, as the pain often prevents use of an extremity. Patients whose pain persists following the healing process of an injury should immediately embark on a regimented physical therapy program. If physical therapy fails and the signs of increased or decreased sympathetic activity are present, a series of pharmacological sympathetic blocks of the extremities should be instituted. Often each block gives progressively longer relief until finally the syndrome abates, although in some patients surgical sympathectomy is necessary. As for any persistent pain syndrome that is difficult to control, multiple other therapies have been proposed, e.g., corticosteroids, vasodilator drugs, tranquilizers, or casting of the involved part. In our experience, these methods usually fail.

POLYCYTHEMIA, MACROGLOBULINS, CRYOPROTEINEMIAS, COLD AGGLUTININS

Some of the factors affecting the rheology of blood may be modified by cold exposure. Patients with cold-precipitable proteins have been well described as exhibiting Raynaud's phenomenon or persistent ischemia probably secondary to rheological abnormalities and occlusion of small blood vessels.

Polycythemia

Brown and Griffin (1930) found that 3 of 100 patients with polycythemia vera manifested attacks of pallor in single digits, and that they were completely relieved by reducing the blood volume. Polycythemia is a cause of the blue toe syndrome, which is actually persistent ischemia.

Walderström's Macroglobulinemia

Imhof and co-workers (1959), in a review of 114 cases of Walderström's macroglobulinemia, reported that 3 percent had Raynaud's phenomenon. If it was due to macroglobulins is questionable, as at least two of these patients also had cryoglobulinemia.

Cryoglobulinemia

Patients with cryoglobulinemia manifest purpura of the lower limbs, arthralgias, leg ulcers, renal failure, and occasionally Raynaud's phenomenon. Essential cryoglobulinemia, without demonstrable underlying disease, usually presents with initial symptoms during the third or fourth decade. It is twice as common in women as in men. Approximately 10 percent have Raynaud's phenomenon. Long-term follow-up has shown that some of these patients develop cirrhosis or lymphoid malignancies (Invernizzi et al., 1983). Secondary cryoglobulinemia may develop in conjunction with infections, autoimmune disorders, or lymphoproliferative diseases. It has been present in patients with Walderström's macroglobulinemia, multiple myeloma, chronic lymphocytic leukemia, Sjögren's syndrome, systemic lupus erythematosus, scleroderma, and liver disease of several etiologies. It has not been found in those with rheumatoid arthritis. Calcinosis cutis, Raynaud's phenomenon, telangiectasia, and thickened, tight skin have been reported in association with primary biliary cirrhosis (Murray-Lyon et al., 1970; Reynolds et al., 1971; Sherlock and Scheuer, 1973) and even in patients with no symptoms of the liver disease (Diederichsen et al., 1981). A common immunological mechanism has been suggested for both diseases. Unfortunately, cryoglobulins were not sought in these patients; high serum immunoglobulin M (IgM) levels are often present.

Pathophysiology

The vascular problems are thought to be produced by precipitation of cryoglobulins at low temperatures. These precipitates behave as immune complexes; activation of the complement pathways may mediate the inflammatory reaction. However, McGrath and Penny (1978) postulated that cryoglobulins impair the peripheral circulation by an increase in blood and plasma viscosity. They found increased plasma and blood viscosity at low shear rates at temperatures of 35° and 25°C in 21 patients with cryoglobulinemia. This increased viscosity correlated with a reduced hand blood flow (plethysmography) measured at 32°, 27°, and 20°C. Imhof and co-workers (1959) noted that cooling of the conjunctiva of one of their patients caused aggregation of erythrocytes and cessation of blood flow within 30 seconds; the stasis lasted 5 minutes following removal of the cold stimulus. A deficiency in sialic acid may alter the solubility of cryoglobulins in the mixed cryoglobulinemias of some of the monoclonal types. The solubility of monoclonal cryoglobulins is thought to involve abnormal amino acid composition or sequences (Zinneman and Caperton, 1977).

Treatment

Successful treatment of symptomatic cryoglobulinemia has been reported with alkylating agents plus prednisone (Ristow et al., 1976). Prednisone alone is usually not of benefit. Melphalan, cyclophosphamide, chlorambucil, and penicillamine have been used. Ristow and co-workers (1976) found that the IgG–IgM cryoprotein levels decreased, but the protein structure was unchanged with melphalan plus prednisone treatment. Plasmapheresis, by removing the circulating cryoprotein, has also relieved symptoms (McLeod and Sassetti, 1980).

Cryofibrinogenemia

Rarely, cryofibrinogens are present in association with cold sensitivity and ischemic lesions of the digits (Ritzmann and Levin, 1961). Jager (1962) reported one patient with Raynaud's phenomenon and sclerodactyly who had a cold precipitate from plasma that was largely fibrinogen.

Cold Agglutinins

Cold agglutinins may also cause cold sensitivity and Raynaud's phenomenon, sometimes with necrosis and gangrene of the fingers, toes, and ears. Pallor or cyanosis often involves the entire hand. The cold agglutinins are most common in patients with virus infections or lymphomas but may occur without apparent cause in elderly patients, inducing cyanosis, hemolytic anemia, and hemoglobinuria

(Ritzmann and Levin, 1961). Men are affected twice as frequently as women in the age group 30 to 90 years (Olesen, 1967). Titers of cold agglutinins are usually higher than 1:128 and consist of antibodies of the γM-immunoglobulin type. Erf (1945) suggested that the thermal range of the antibody was important for determining the severity of the disease, as the clinical picture is not always related to the titers. The vascular problems are believed due to intravascular clumping of red blood cells, with a marked decrease in blood flow in small vessels (Hansen and Faber, 1947). Cooling the conjunctiva in patients causes a reversible hemagglutination of red blood cells with cessation of blood flow in the visualized blood vessels (Nelson and Marshall, 1953). However, other observers hypothesized that an associated vasospastic condition contributed to the reduction in blood flow (Carey et al., 1948; Kramer and Perilstein, 1951). Marshall and co-workers (1953) studied hand (plethysmography) and finger (calorimetry) blood flows in two patients. During local exposure to 10°C or colder water, blood flow in the hand was arrested and the fingers failed to show cold vasodilatation (see Fig. 1–8). These findings were in contrast to the maintenance of blood flow and cold vasodilatation in patients with primary Raynaud's disease under similar circumstances. Hillestad (1959) confirmed these findings and showed that nerve blocks, which inhibit sympathetic nerves, delayed but did not prevent the arrest of hand blood flow (plethysmography). Both groups of investigators concluded that the Raynaud's phenomenon could be explained by a mechanical obstruction of the vessels by agglutinated red blood cells and that it was unnecessary to postulate a vasospastic component.

Treatment of patients with cold agglutinins and vascular manifestations has depended on the avoidance of cold stimulation. Chlorambucil reduces the quantity of cold agglutinins, but it is a toxic drug that must be given for prolonged periods (Olesen, 1967).

Summary

It may be concluded that cryoproteinemias are a rare cause of Raynaud's phenomenon. Many patients with cryoglobulins, cryofibrinogens, or cold agglutinins are asymptomatic. Some other factor may be necessary to produce the vasospastic attacks. Because men are affected more often than women, it is unlikely that these patients have underlying primary Raynaud's disease. Patients with polycythemia may also develop Raynaud's phenomenon, but a persistent digital ischemia is more common. Macroglobulins without cryoproteins are a doubtful cause of Raynaud's phenomenon.

VINYL CHLORIDE DISEASE

Raynaud's phenomenon is a common occurrence in patients with vinyl chloride disease. Exposure to vinyl chloride may cause a multisystem disease that can resemble scleroderma in that there is thickening of the skin of the hands and forearms with nodule formation, and acroosteolysis occurs. Thrombocytopenia, portal fibrosis, hepatic and pulmonary dysfunction, and angiosarcomas of the liver have been described.

Exposure and Incidence

Polyvinyl chloride plastics are made by polymerization from vinyl chloride gas. The disease has been reported mostly in workers who clean the autoclaves, although the baggers also have an increased incidence. The substance causing the disease is unknown, as it may be a by-product of the vinyl chloride. The incidence of symptomatic disease in the workers has been estimated at 3 percent or less (Markowitz et al., 1972).

Pathophysiology

Circulating immune complexes have been found in more than 60 percent of symptomatic patients but in few asymptomatic workers (Ward et al., 1976). There is a polyclonal increase of one of the immunoglobulins, usually IgG; mixed cryoglobulins and an abnormal conversion of complement fractions C4 and C3 are also seen. The antinuclear antibody test may be positive in low titers (Johnston, 1978; Ward et al., 1976). Immunofluorescence studies of skin biopsies have shown aggregates of IgG, C4, C3, fibrinogen, and fibrin in the lumens of vessels and adherent to the endothelium. These substances were also detected in the media and subintimal regions of small and medium-sized arterioles. Langauer-Lewowicka and co-workers (1976) detected a latent cryoglobulinemia in 82 percent of their patients by Sephadex G-200 filtration and considered that it was pathogenetically important.

Pathology

Widefield capillary microscopy of the fingernail beds has demonstrated dilated capillary loops, short capillaries, disarrangement of capillary polarity, and avascular areas that resemble a scleroderma pattern but in scattered areas in approximately 40 percent of unselected workers (Langauer-Lewowicka, 1983; Maricq et al., 1976). These changes did not correlate with length of exposure, age, or tobacco smoking. Angiography has revealed segmental occlusions or stenoses of digital arteries with extensive collateralization; elongation and tortuosity of the digital arteries may occur (Falappa et al., 1982; Johnston, 1978; Koischwitz et al., 1980). Skin biopsies have revealed a thickened dermis, nonfibrillary homogenization of collagen, and thickened, swollen collagen (Markowitz et al., 1972). Lymphocytes, histiocytes, and disorganized elastic fibers are also present.

Bone Involvement

In addition to Raynaud's phenomenon, osteolysis may occur. Radiography may show dissolution of central parts of the terminal phalanges, periarticular erosions of the finger joints, and erosions of the terminal phalanges (Harris and Adams,

1967; Johnston, 1978; Markowitz et al., 1972). Actually, these changes have been described in many other bones of the body as well. Harris and Adams (1967) found only two cases of acroosteolysis after screening 588 workers in a polyvinyl chloride factory.

Treatment

Removing the patient from exposure to the chemicals usually results in a gradual improvement in the thickened skin, but the bony changes may continue. Information is not available regarding the prognosis for the Raynaud's phenomenon.

Summary

A few vinyl chloride workers, especially those who clean the vats, may develop Raynaud's phenomenon as part of a systemic disease. Abnormalities in immunoglobulins and the complement system may be present; dermal collagen appears to be involved. Digital artery obstructive disease and capillary loop dilatations are common. Treatment involves removing the patient from the toxic environment.

NEOPLASMS

Patients with a variety of neoplastic diseases may develop Raynaud's phenomenon or digital ischemia. Such occurrences are usually due to cryoglobulinemia, compression of the cervical sympathetic chain, carpal tunnel syndrome, or cold agglutinins. However, some patients have none of these abnormalities. Hawley and co-workers (1967) reported that four of six patients with digital ischemia and tumors had no underlying abnormalities to explain the ischemia. All the patients were female, the youngest being 42 years old. Cancer of the stomach, kidney, colon, and ovary were represented. Friedman and co-workers (1969) reported two cases of cancer (cervix and breast) and digital ischemia; occlusion of the popliteal arteries was found in one case. Histology of the digital vessels in one of these patients revealed fibrinoid necrosis, intimal proliferation, and moderate inflammatory cell infiltration suggesting a vasculitis. Powell (1973) reported a case of severe Raynaud's phenomenon and digital gangrene preceding the discovery of acute lymphatic leukemia; the patient was a 7-year-old boy. Palmer and Vedi (1974) found no dysproteinemias in three elderly women with Raynaud's phenomenon and reticulum cell sarcoma, cancer of the stomach, and cancer of the stomach or pancreas.

Andrasch and co-workers (1976) described digital ischemia in a patient with a sarcomatoid adenocarcinoma of the kidney and a high level of gamma globulins. Skin biopsy of the forearm showed mild leukocytoclastic angiitis, and an arteriogram showed digital arterial irregularities and narrowings unresponsive to intraarterial reserpine. Immunofluorescence of the tumor showed substantial deposits of IgG lining the tumor cells, and electron microscopy revealed dense deposits in the endothelium of small arteries. Andrasch et al. suggested that antibodies to tumor antigens may have been involved as the cause of the Raynaud's phenomenon.

Wytock and colleagues (1983) described Raynaud's phenomenon of 2 years' duration in a 59-year-old woman that resolved with resection of a small bowel adenocarcinoma and was still absent 5 years later. No cryglobulins were present. These authors reviewed 180 cases of malignancy associated with Raynaud's phenomenon seen over a 6-year period at the Mayo Clinic. In 63 cases the vasospastic disease preceded the tumor discovery by an average of 9.8 years. Breast and lung cancer were the most frequent, and no cases resolved after resection of the tumor. No information is given regarding the blood status or metastases in these patients.

Taylor and co-workers (1987) described five patients who had Raynaud's phenomenon and malignancy (breast, gastric, and renal tumors and leukemia). These patients were considered to have digital artery obstructions due to hyperviscosity, arteritis, or a hypercoagulable state.

It can be concluded that Raynaud's phenomenon or digital ischemia may be a rare manifestation of malignancies of many varieties and is most common in women, even in the absence of dysproteinemias or involvement of the cervical sympathetic nerves. So far the cause is unknown, although a vasculitis or hypercoagulable state are primary suspects.

HYPOTHYROIDISM

Raynaud's phenomenon has been reported in patients with hypothyroidism, with alleviation of the vasospastic attacks after thyroid replacement. Shagan and Friedman described two patients with hypothyroidism (1976) and one with panhypopituitarism (1980) who had Raynaud's phenomenon. After thyroid replacement therapy, the phenomenon disappeared within 1 to 4 months, although the hands remained cool and hyperhidrotic in a warm environment. Nielsen and co-workers (1982) studied 17 patients with myxedema; four patients had Raynaud's phenomenon (24 percent), and 15 had cold hands (88 percent). These authors found an abnormal finger systolic pressure with 10°C local cooling in 8 of the 17 patients that improved significantly during thyroid treatment. They did not consider the frequency of Raynaud's phenomenon to be increased compared to a young female population. Because the patients responded to thyroid therapy, they postulated that Raynaud's phenomenon may occur in a group of hypothyroid patients who were predisposed to the disease.

The blood flow in the extremities of patients with myxedema has been shown to be decreased (Stewart and Evans, 1942). The decreased heat production of these patients may produce peripheral vasoconstriction in an attempt to conserve body heat, and the increased sympathetic nerve activity may explain the increased plasma norepinephrine concentrations found in myxedematous patients (Christensen, 1973). Hypothyroid rats have been shown to be hypersensitive to the vasoconstrictor action of norepinephrine (Koehn et al., 1967). It is also possible that thickening of the vascular wall by edema could lead to closure of the vessels with normal sympathetic stimuli.

It can be concluded that patients with hypothyroidism have cold extremities and that some develop Raynaud's phenomenon. It is probably a separate etiology of the phenomenon, as it responds to thyroid replacement. However, it is of interest that Peacock (1960) reported successfully treating primary Raynaud's disease with thyroid preparations.

HEPATITIS B ANTIGENEMIA

A vasculitis (periarteritis nodosa or necrotizing vasculitis) with hypertension, arthritis, neuropathy, pericarditis, renal disease, and skin rash has been associated with hepatitis B virus (Gocke et al., 1970). Raynaud's phenomenon may be part of this syndrome. Kim and Koff (1974) described a man who had had Raynaud's phenomenon for 20 years and asymptomatic chronic active hepatitis with circulating hepatitis B antigen. No other cause for the vasospastic syndrome was found, and the patient became asymptomatic with prednisone and phenoxybenzamine therapy. Cosgriff and Arnold (1976) reported a patient who manifested fever, arthralgias, and Raynaud's phenomenon with infections of the fingertips; the test for hepatitis B antigen was positive. Icteric hepatitis manifested 1 month later. The finger lesions resolved by the time the hepatitis became apparent clinically. McMahon and co-workers (1980) described six cases of hepatitis B-associated vasculitis; all six patients tested positive for the hepatitis B surface antigen, and the five tested had hepatitis Be antigen as well. Two of the six patients had Raynaud's phenomenon. Biopsy showed mononuclear infiltrates and fibrinoid necrosis of small arteries and arterioles of the skin, muscle, and nerve.

Thus hepatitis B may be a rare cause of Raynaud's phenomenon. A vasculitis manifested with Raynaud's phenomenon alone or with other organ involvement may occur during the prodrome or after the development of hepatitis that is hepatitis B antigen-positive. The vasculitis and Raynaud's phenomenon may improve and even disappear with steroid therapy (Cosgriff and Arnold, 1976; Kim and Koff, 1974).

MISCELLANEOUS ETIOLOGIES

Intraarterial Injections

Unilateral extremity vasospasm often progressing to gangrene has been reported after intraarterial injection of drugs. The offending agents have included barbiturate preparations, meperidine, promazine, ether, amphetamine, sodium sulfobromophthalein, and street drugs (Engler et al., 1967; Hager et al., 1967). Most of these cases are due to inadvertent intraarterial administration in the upper extremity (the artery lies close to the vein in the antecubital fossa). A concentrated solution of the drug is then delivered to the digital arterial tree.

The injection is usually followed by immediate pain in the arm and hand, and the hand and fingers become mottled blue and cold. This phase may be followed by edema of the forearm and hand and then gangrene of the fingers and hand. Distal pulses may be present but may disappear later. Angiography usually reveals severe vasospasm of the arteries of the forearm, hand, and fingers; radial or ulnar artery occlusions may be present (Singer, 1976).

Engler and co-workers (1964) have studied the pathogenesis and pathology in dogs. Three hours after intraarterial injections of various drugs, inflammatory changes appeared in the small blood vessels and later in the larger arteries. It resulted in extravasation of blood, vessel wall necrosis, and thrombosis. Because some patients maintain normal distal large-vessel pulses, most of the injury is thought to occur in the small vessels.

Treatment is usually unsatisfactory. Anticoagulation, sympathectomy, and thrombectomy have been used. Intermittent positive pressure applied to the affected part may control the edema and obviate the need for a fasciotomy (Engler et al., 1967). Many cases progress to gangrene, but in a few patients the symptoms resolve slowly with no breakdown of tissue.

The primary aim of prophylaxis must be to avoid intraarterial injections. Tourniquets should not be applied too tightly during intravenous injections. The syringe should be watched carefully for pulsatile flow after insertion of the needle.

Arteriovenous Fistula

More than 50 percent of patients with A-V fistulas may develop Raynaud's phenomenon; it is most common in patients undergoing hemodialysis (Lappchen et al., 1977; Nielsen and Lokkegaard, 1981). Diminished blood flow occurs distal to a fistula, and peripheral coldness and trophic changes may occur (Wakim and Jones, 1958). Blood pressure in the fingers is significantly lower in the arm with the fistula than in the other arm, and abnormal closure of the digital arteries occurs with 15°C cooling (Nielsen and Lokkegaard, 1981). However, this reaction was also found in the fingers of the opposite hand, indicating that the cold sensitivity may not be due entirely to the large increase in forearm blood flow and decrease in finger blood flow. Patients do have increased norepinephrine levels during dialysis, so that increased sympathetic nervous system activity may be at fault. Renal transplantation has been reported to improve the cold sensitivity (Lappchen et al., 1977).

Renal Disease

Patient with severe renal disease have also been described as having marked calcification of their medium-sized and digital arteries. They may have cool, cyanotic hands, and gangrene may occur. There is no predilection for sex or age, or for a specific type of renal disease. The pathogenesis of the ischemia is not known, as extensive medial calcification occurs with other diseases and in renal patients without vasospastic changes or gangrene; moreover, in some patients the skin lesions heal soon after parathyroidectomy, before the calcification can regress. Mechanical obstruction due to calcium deposition, parathormone, hypercalcemia, and steroid or immunosuppressive agents has been suggested as important in the etiology (Gipstein et al., 1976). This calcification can often be palpated in the medium-sized arteries; occasionally all subcutaneous vessels can be felt by palpating the skin. The arterial calcifications can be seen by radiography of the areas involved. Arteriography in one patient showed occlusion of both the radial and the ulnar arteries. Biopsies exhibit marked medial and intimal calcification with narrowing of the arterial lumen, and immunoglobulins have not been found (Friedman et al., 1969; Gipstein et al., 1976). The arterial calcification is probably due to secondary hyperparathyroidism; phosphorus and calcium blood levels may be elevated. Some patients respond to parathyroidectomy.

Unknown Etiology and Vasculitis

Despite the advent of more accurate tests for the diagnosis of underlying diseases, groups of patients with vasospastic disease of the hands and fingers of unknown origin continue to be described (Bauer et al., 1977; Rowell, 1977). The patients have had extensive work-ups for secondary diseases. In these patients, who often present with acute onset of ischemia of the hands, there may be diffuse obstruction of the palmar arches and the digital, radial, or ulnar arteries. Biopsies have revealed thrombosis or fibrotic obliteration of the ulnar artery; endarteritis without immune complexes was reported in one patient. Fingertip ulcers and gangrene may occur. One study reported that the problem was not recurrent (Bauer et al., 1977).

Blunt and Porter (1981) reported that 26 of 141 patients with Raynaud's phenomenon had a suspected vasculitis. However, these patients had systemic symptoms, and tests for antinuclear antibodies or rheumatoid factor were frequently positive. Their disease probably should be classified as a connective tissue disorder. Raynaud's phenomenon does occur in patients with vasculitis and is due to several causes (discussed in this chapter), including connective tissue diseases, cryoglobulinemia, vinyl chloride disease, and hepatitis B antigenemia. These patients may have immune complexes, which can induce an inflammatory reaction in small blood vessels, but the relation to the development of cold sensitivity is unknown.

Heavy Metals

Intoxication with heavy metals such as lead, arsenic, thallium, and mercury has been mentioned as a cause of Raynaud's phenomenon. There is little substantiation, however, that these substances cause episodic, well-demarcated vasospastic attacks.

REFERENCES

Blunt RJ, Porter JM: Raynaud's syndrome. *Semin Arthritis Rheumatol* 10:282, 1981.
Jeune R, Thivolet J: Etude arteriographique de la main au cours de 52 phenomenes de Raynaud d'etiologie diverse. *Nouv Presse Med* 7:2619, 1978.

β-Adrenoceptor Blocking Drugs
Bolli P, Waal-Manning HJ, Simpson FO, Seeman IHM: Treatment of hypertension with labetalol. *NZ Med J* 86:557, 1977.

Coffman JD, Rasmussen HM: Effects of β-adrenoceptor blocking drugs in patients with Raynaud's phenomenon. *Circulation* 72:466, 1985.

Cohen RA, Coffman JD: β-Adrenergic vasodilator mechanism in the finger. *Circ Res* 49:1196, 1981.

Eliasson K, Lins L, Sundqvist K: Vasospastic phenomena in patients treated with beta-adrenoceptor blocking agents. *Acta Med Scand* [Suppl] 628:39, 1979.

Eliasson K, Lins L, Sundqvist K: Peripheral vasospasm during β-receptor blockade—a comparison between metoprolol and pindolol. *Acta Med Scand* [Suppl] 665:109, 1982.

Eliasson K, Danielson M, Hylander B, Lindblad LE: Raynaud's phenomenon caused by β-receptor blocking drugs. *Acta Med Scand* 215:333, 1984.

Erb RJ, Plachetka JR: Thermographic evaluation of the peripheral vascular effects of labetalol and propranolol. *Curr Ther Res* 38:68, 1985.

Feleke E, Lyngstam O, Rastam L, Ryden L: Complaints of cold extremities among patients on antihypertensive treatment. *Acta Med Scand* 213:381, 1983.

Frohlich ED, Tarazi RC, Dunstan HP: Peripheral arterial insufficiency. *JAMA* 208:2471, 1969.

Heck I, Trubestein G, Stumpe KO: Effects of combined β- and α-receptor blockade on peripheral circulation in essential hypertension. *Clin Sci* 61:429s, 1981.

Holti G: A comparison of two beta-blocking drugs in patients with Raynaud's phenomenon. *Practitioner* 226:781, 1982.

Lenders JWM, Salemans J, de Boo T, Lemmens WAJ, Thien T, van't Laar A: The influence of intrinsic sympathomimetic activity and beta-1 receptor selectivity on the recovery of finger skin temperature after finger cooling in normotensive subjects. *Clin Pharmacol Ther* 39:353, 1986.

Marshall AJ, Roberts CJC, Barritt DW: Raynaud's phenomenon as side effect of beta-blockers in hypertension. *Br Med J* 1:1498, 1976.

McSorley PD, Warren DJ: Effects of propranolol and metoprolol on the peripheral circulation. *Br Med J* 2:1598, 1978.

Medical Research Council Working Party on Mild to Moderate Hypertension: Adverse reactions to bendrofluazide and propranolol for the treatment of mild hypertension. *Lancet* 2:539, 1981.

Nielsen PE, Nielsen SL: Digital arterial tone in hypertensive subjects treated with cardioselective and non-selective beta-adrenoreceptor blocking agents. *Dan Med Bull* 28:76, 1981.

Nielsen SL, Olsen N, Nielsen PE: Increased digital arterial tone in hypertensive subjects indicated by local cooling and propranolol treatment. *Clin Physiol* 1:21, 1981.

Steiner JA, Cooper R, Gear JS, Ledingham JGG: Vascular symptoms in patients with primary Raynaud's phenomenon are not exacerbated by propranolol or labetalol. *Br J Clin Pharmacol* 7:401, 1979.

Steiner JA, Cooper R, McPherson K, Riley AJ: Effect of β-adrenoceptor antagonists on prevalence of peripheral vascular symptoms in hypertensive patients. *Br J Clin Pharmacol* 14:833, 1982.

Vale JA, Jefferys DB: Peripheral gangrene complicating beta-blockade. *Lancet* 1:1216, 1978.

VandenBurg MJ, Cooper WD, Woollard ML, Currie WJC, Bowker CH: Reduced peripheral vascular symptoms in elderly patients treated with α-methyldopa—a comparison with propranolol. *Eur J Clin Pharmacol* 26:325, 1984a.

VandenBurg MJ, Evans SJW, Cooper WD, Bradshaw F, Currie WJC: Is the feeling of cold extremities experienced by hypertensive patients due to their disease or their treatment? *Eur J Clin Pharmacol* 27:47, 1984b.

Van der Veur E, ten Berge BS, Wouda AA, Wesseling H: Effects of atenolol, labetalol and propranolol on the peripheral circulation in hypertensive patients without obstructive vascular disease. *Eur J Clin Pharmacol* 28:131, 1985.

White C de B, Udwadia BP: β-Adrenoceptors in the human dorsal hand vein, and the effects of propranolol and practolol on venous sensitivity to noradrenaline. *Br J Clin Pharmacol* 2:99, 1975.

Wollersheim H, Lenders J, Peters H, Thien T: Influence of cold challenge on finger skin temperature during long-term use of beta-adrenoceptor blocking drugs in hypertensive patients. *Int Angiol* 6:307, 1987.

Zacharias FJ: Patient acceptability of propranolol and occurrence of side effects. *Postgrad Med J* 52(suppl 4):87, 1976.

Ergot Preparations

Aellig WH: Influence of ergot compounds on compliance of superficial hand veins in man. *Postgrad Med J* 52(suppl 1):21, 1976.

Bagby RJ, Cooper RD: Angiography in ergotism. *AJR* 116:179, 1972.

Bluntschli HJ, Goetz RH: The effect of ergot derivatives on the circulation in man with special reference to two new hydrogenated compounds (dihydroergotamine and dihydroergocornine) *Am Heart J* 35:873, 1948.

Brismar B, Somell A, Lockner D: Arterial insufficiency caused by ergotism. *Acta Chir Scand* 143:319, 1977.

Cameron EA, French EB: St. Anthony's fire rekindled: gangrene due to therapeutic dose of ergotamine. *Br Med J* 2:28, 1960.

Carliner NH, Denune DP, Finch CS Jr, Goldberg LI: Sodium nitroprusside treatment of ergotamine-induced peripheral ischemia. *JAMA* 227:308, 1974.

Cobaugh DS: Prazosin treatment of ergotamine-induced peripheral ischemia. *JAMA* 244:1360, 1980.

Dagher FJ, Pais SO, Richards W, Queral LA: Severe unilateral ischemia of the lower extremity caused by ergotamine: treatment with nifedipine. *Surgery* 97:369, 1985.

Dierckx RA, Peters O, Ebinger G, Six R, Corne L: Intraarterial sodium nitroprusside infusion in the treatment of severe ergotism. *Clin Neuropharmacol* 9:542, 1986.

Dige-Petersen H, Lassen NA, Noer I, Tonnesen KH: Subclinical ergotism. *Lancet* 2:65, 1977.

Greenberg DJ, Hallett JW Jr: Lower extremity ischemia due to combined drug therapy for migraine. *Postgrad Med* 72:103, 1982.

Greene FL, Ariyan S, Stansel HC Jr: Mesenteric and peripheral vascular ischemia secondary to ergotism. *Surgery* 81:176, 1977.

Herlache J, Hoskins P, Schmidt CM: Ergotism. *Angiology* 24:369, 1973.

Hessov I, Kromann-Andersen C, Madsen B: Peripheral arterial insufficiency during ergotamine treatment. *Dan Med Bull* 19:236, 1972.

Husted JW, Ring EJ, Hirsh LF: Intraarterial nitroprusside treatment for ergotism. *AJR* 131:1090, 1978.

Husum B, Metz P, Rasmussen JP: Nitroglycerin infusion for ergotism. *Lancet* 2:794, 1979.

Innes IR: Identification of the smooth muscle excitatory receptor for ergot alkaloids. *Br J Pharmacol* 19:120, 1962.

Kaunitz J: Chronic endemic ergotism. *Arch Surg* 25:1135, 1932.

Kemerer VF, Dagher FJ, Pais SO: Successful treatment of ergotism with nifedipine. *AJR* 143:333, 1984.

Kempczinski RF, Buckley CV, Darling RC: Vascular insufficiency secondary to ergotism. *Surgery* 79:597, 1976.

Lewis T: The manner in which necrosis arises in the fowl's comb under ergot poisoning. *Clin Sci* 2:43, 1935.

Muller-Schweinitzer E: Responsiveness of isolated canine cerebral and peripheral arteries to ergotamine. *Arch Pharmacol* 292:113, 1976.

O'Dell CW Jr, Davis GB, Johnson AD, Safdi MA, Brant-Zawadzki M, Bookstein JJ: Sodium nitroprusside in the treatment of ergotism. *Radiology* 124:73, 1977.

Shifrin E, Perel A, Olschwang D, Diamant Y, Cotev S: Reversal of ergotamine-induced arteriospasm by mechanical intra-arterial dilatation. *Lancet* 2:1278, 1980.

Tfelt-Hansen P, Ostergaard JR, Gothgen I, Jacobsen E, Rasmussen JP, Husum B: Nitroglycerin for ergotism: experimental studies in vitro and in migraine patients and treatment of an overt case. *Eur J Clin Pharmacol* 22:105, 1982.

Young JR, Humphries AW: Severe arteriospasm after use of ergotamine tartrate suppositories. *JAMA* 175:1141, 1961.

Zimran A, Ofek B, Hershko C: Treatment with captopril for peripheral ischemia induced by ergotamine. *Br Med J* 1:288, 1984.

Methysergide

Ameli FM, Nathanson M, Elkan I: Methysergide therapy causing vascular insufficiency of the upper limb. *Can J Surg* 20:158, 1977.

Graham JR: Methysergide for prevention of headache. *N Engl J Med* 270:67, 1964.

Johnson TD: Severe peripheral arterial constriction, acute ischemia of lower extremity with use of methysergide and ergotamine. *Arch Intern Med* 117:237, 1966.

Vinblastine and Bleomycin

Chernicoff DP, Bukowski RM, Young JR: Raynaud's phenomenon after bleomycin treatment. *Cancer Treat Rep* 62:570, 1978.

Cohen IS, Mosher MB, O'Keefe EJ, Klaus SN, DeConti RC: Cutaneous toxicity of bleomycin therapy. *Arch Dermatol* 107:553, 1973.

Elomaa I, Pajunen M, Virkkunen P: Raynaud's phenomenon progressing to gangrene after vincristine and bleomycin therapy. *Acta Med Scand* 216:323, 1984.

Grau JJ, Grau M, Milla A, Estape J, Mulet M: Cancer chemotherapy and Raynaud's phenomenon. *Ann Intern Med* 98:258, 1983.

Kukla LJ, McGuire WP, Lad T, Saltiel M: Acute vascular episodes associated with therapy for carcinomas of the upper aerodigestive tract with bleomycin, vincristine, and cisplatin. *Cancer Treat Rep* 66:369, 1982.

Rothberg H: Raynaud's phenomenon after vinblastine-bleomycin chemotherapy. *Cancer Treat Rep* 62:569, 1978.

Scheulen ME, Schmidt CG: Raynaud's phenomenon and cancer chemotherapy. *Ann Intern Med* 96:256, 1982.

Soble AR: Chronic bleomycin-associated Raynaud's phenomenon. *Cancer Treat Rep* 62:570, 1978.

Teutsch C, Lipton A, Harvey HA: Raynaud's phenomenon as a side effect of chemotherapy with vinblastine and bleomycin for testicular carcinoma. *Cancer Treat Rep* 61:925, 1977.

Vogelzang NJ, Bosl GJ, Johnson K, Kennedy BJ: Raynaud's phenomenon: a common toxicity after combination chemotherapy for testicular cancer. *Ann Intern Med* 95:288, 1981.

Nitroglycerin, Amphetamines, Imipramine

Applebaum PS, Kapoor W: Imipramine-induced vasospasm: a case report. *Am J Psychiatry* 140:913, 1983.

Bower JS, Davis GB, Kearney TE, Bardin J: Diffuse vascular spasm associated with 4-bromo-2,5 dimethoxyamphetamine ingestion. *JAMA* 249:1477, 1983.

Lange RL, Reid MS, Tresch DD, Keelan MH, Bernhard VM, Coolidge G: Nonatheromatous ischemic heart disease following withdrawal from chronic industrial nitroglycerin exposure. *Circulation* 46:666, 1972.

Cyclosporin

Deray G, LeHoang P, Achour L, Hornych A, Landault C, Caraillon A: Cyclosporin and Raynaud phenomenon. *Lancet* 3:1092, 1986.

Oral Contraceptives

Birnstingl M: The Raynaud syndrome. *Postgrad Med J* 47:297, 1971.
Bole GG Jr, Friedlsender MH, Smith CK: Rheumatic symptoms and serological abnormalities induced by oral contraceptives. *Lancet* 1:323, 1969.

Connective Tissue Diseases

Boylan RC, Sokoloff L: Vascular lesions in dermatomyositis. *Arthritis Rheum* 3:379, 1960.
Coffman JD: Skin blood flow in scleroderma. *J Lab Clin Med* 76: 480, 1970.
Dimant J, Ginzler E, Schlesinger M, Sterba G, Diamond H, Kaplan D, Weiner M: The clinical significance of Raynaud's phenomenon in systemic lupus erythematosus. *Arthritis Rheum* 22:815, 1979.
Ellman MH, Pachman L, Medof ME: Raynaud's phenomenon and initially seronegative mixed connective tissue disease. *J Rheumatol* 8:632, 1981.
Estes D, Christian CL: The natural history of systemic lupus erythematosus by prospective analysis. *Medicine* 50:85, 1971.
Farmer RG, Gifford RW, Hines EA: Raynaud's disease with sclerodactylia. *Circulation* 23:13, 1961.
Fessel WJ: Systemic lupus erythematosus in the community. *Arch Intern Med* 134: 1027, 1974.
Fox RI, Howell FV, Bone RC, Michelson P: Primary Sjögren syndrome: clinical and immunopathologic features. *Semin Arthritis Rheum* 14:77, 1984.
Fries JF: Physiologic studies in systemic sclerosis (scleroderma). *Arch Intern Med* 123:22, 1969.
Fritzler MJ, Kinsella TD: The CREST syndrome: a distinct serologic entity with anticentromere antibodies. *Am J Med* 69:520, 1980.
Harvey AM, Schulman LE, Tumulty PA, Conly CL, Schoenreich EH: Raynaud's phenomenon associated with lupus erythematosus: review of the literature and clinical analysis of 138 cases. *Medicine* 33:291, 1954.
Hochberg MC, Boyd RE, Ahearn JM, Arnett FC, Bias WB, Provost TT, Stevens MB: Systemic lupus erythematosus: a review of clinico-laboratory features and immunogenetic markers in 150 patients with emphasis on demographic subsets. *Medicine* 64:285, 1985.
Hostein J, Bost R, Carpentier P, Franco A, Fournet J: Motricite oesophagienne au cours de la maladie de Raynaud, de la sclerodermie systemique et du syndrome de Raynaud presclerodermique. *Gastroenterol Clin Biol* 9:130, 1985.
Jablonska S: *Scleroderma and Pseudoscleroderma.* Warshaw: Polish Medical Publications, 1965.
Johansson EA, Niemi K-M, Lassus A, Gripenberg M: Mixed connective tissue disease: a followup study of 12 patients with special reference to cold sensitivity and skin manifestations. *Acta Dermatovener* (Stockh) 61:225, 1981.
Kenamore BD, Levin WC, Ritzmann SE: Raynaud's phenomenon as leading sign of lupus erythematosus—report of three cases and classification of cryopathies. *Texas Reports Biol Med* 26:189, 1968.
Laws JW, Lillie JG, Scott JT: Arteriographic appearance in rheumatoid arthritis and other disorders. *Br J Radiol* 36:477, 1963.
LeRoy EC, Downey JA, Cannon PJ: Skin capillary blood flow in scleroderma. *J Clin Invest* 50:930, 1971.

LeRoy EC, Black C, Fleischmajer R, Jablonska S, Krieg T, Medsger TA Jr, Rowell N, Wollheim F: Scleroderma (systemic sclerosis): classification, subsets, and pathogenesis. *J Rheumatol* 15:202, 1988.

Masi AT, Rodnan GP: Preliminary criteria for the classification of systemic sclerosis (scleroderma). *Arthritis Rheum* 23:581, 1980.

Nimelstein SH, Brody S, McShane D, Holman HR: Mixed connective tissue disease: a subsequent evaluation of the original 25 patients. *Medicine* 59:239, 1980.

Reeves WH, Fisher DE, Wisniewolski R, Gottlieb AB, Chiorazzi N: Psoriasis and Raynaud's phenomenon associated with autoantibodies to U1 and U2 small nuclear ribonucleoproteins. *N Engl J Med* 315:105, 1986.

Sapira JD, Rodnan GP, Scheib ET, Klaniecki T, Rizk M: Studies of endogenous catecholamines in patients with Raynaud's phenomenon secondary to progressive systemic sclerosis (scleroderma). *Am J Med* 52:330, 1972.

Scott JT, Hourihane DO, Doyle FH, Steiner RE, Laws JW, Dixon AStJ, Bywaters EGL: Digital arteries in rheumatoid disease. *Ann Rheum Dis* 20:224, 1961.

Sharp GC: Mixed connective tissue disease. *Bull Rheum Dis* 25:828, 1975.

Smith FE, Sweet DE, Brunner CM, Davis JS: Avascular necrosis in SLE: an apparent predilection for younger patients. *Ann Rheum Dis* 35:227, 1976.

Sodeman W, Burch G: Tissue pressure: an objective method of following skin changes in scleroderma. *Am Heart J* 17:21, 1939.

Tan EM, Rodnan GP, Garcia I, Moroi Y, Fritzler MJ, Peebles C: Diversity of antinuclear antibodies in progressive systemic sclerosis: anti-centromere antibody and its relationship to CREST syndrome. *Arthritis Rheum* 23:617, 1980.

Tan EM, Cohen AS, Fries JF, Masi AT, McShane DJ, Rothfield NF, Schaller JG, Talal N, Winchester RJ: The 1982 revised criteria for the classification of systemic lupus erythematosus. *Arthritis Rheum* 25:1271, 1982.

Thibierge G, Weissenbach RJ: Concretion calcanes sous cutanees et sclerodermie. *Ann Dermatol Syph* 2:129, 1911.

Tuffanelli DL, Dubois EL: Cutaneous manifestations of systemic lupus erythematosus. *Arch Dermatol* 90:377, 1964.

Tuffanelli DL, Winkelmann RK: Systemic scleroderma: a clinical study of 727 cases. *Arch Dermatol* 84:359, 1961.

Primary Pulmonary Hypertension

Celoria GC, Friedell GH, Sommers SC: Raynaud's disease and primary pulmonary hypertension. *Circulation* 22:1055, 1960.

Fahey PJ, Utell MJ, Condemi JJ, Green R, Hyde RW: Raynaud's phenomenon of the lung. *Am J Med* 76:263, 1984.

Fisher J, Mack RJ, Likier HM, Schiff AN, Borer JS: Nifedipine in pulmonary arterial hypertension: importance of Raynaud's phenomenon. *Chest* 92:400, 1987.

Fuster V, Steele PM, Edwards WD, Gersh BJ, McGoon MD, Frye RL: Primary pulmonary hypertension: natural history and the importance of thrombosis. *Circulation* 70:580, 1984.

Miller MJ: Effect of the cold pressor test on diffusing capacity. *Chest* 84:264, 1983.

Shuck JW, Oetgen WJ, Tesar JT: Pulmonary vascular response during Raynaud's phenomenon in progressive systemic sclerosis. *Am J Med* 78:221, 1985.

Smith WM, Kroop IG: Raynaud's disease in primary pulmonary hypertension. *JAMA* 165:1245, 1957.

Walcott G, Burchell HB, Brown AL: Primary pulmonary hypertension. *Am J Med* 49:70, 1970.

Winters WL, Joseph RR, Learner N: "Primary" pulmonary hypertension and Raynaud's phenomenon. *Arch Intern Med* 114:821, 1964.

Wise RA, Wigley F, Newball HH, Stevens MB: The effect of cold exposure on diffusing capacity in patients with Raynaud's phenomenon. *Chest* 81:695, 1982.

Traumatic Vasospastic Disease

Ashe WF, Cook WT, Old JW: Raynaud's phenomenon of occupational origin. *Arch Environ Health* 5:333, 1962.

Azuma T, Ohhashi T, Sakaguchi M: Vibration-induced hyperresponsiveness of arterial smooth muscle to noradrenaline with special reference to Raynaud's phenomenon in vibration disease. *Cardiovasc Res* 12:758, 1978.

Azuma T, Ohhashi T, Sakaguchi M: An approach to the pathogenesis of "white finger" induced by vibratory stimulation: acute but sustained changes in vascular responsiveness of canine hindlimb to noradrenaline. *Cardiovasc Res* 14:725, 1980.

Banister PA, Smith FV: Vibration-induced white fingers and manipulative dexterity. *Br J Industr Med* 29:264, 1972.

Bovenzi M: Some pathophysiological aspects of vibration-induced white finger. *Eur J Appl Physiol* 55:381, 1986.

Chatterjee DS, Petrie A, Taylor W: Prevalence of vibration-induced white finger in fluorspar mines in Weardale. *Br J Industr Med* 35:208, 1978.

Ekenvall L, Carlson A: Vibration white finger: a follow up study. *Br J Industr Med* 44:476, 1987.

Ekenvall L, Lindblad LE: Vibration white finger and digital systolic pressure during cooling. *Br J Industr Med* 43:280, 1986a.

Ekenvall L, Lindblad LE: Is vibration white finger a primary sympathetic nerve injury? *Br J Industr Med* 43:702, 1986b.

Farkkila M, Pyykko I: Blood flow in the contralateral hand during vibration and hand grip contractions of lumberjacks. *Scand J Work Environ Health* 5:368, 1979.

Futatsuka M: Epidemiological studies of vibration disease due to brush saw operation. *Int Arch Occup Environ Health* 54:251, 1984.

Futatsuka M, Ueno T: Vibration exposure and vibration-induced white finger due to chain saw operation. *J Occup Med* 27:257, 1985.

Futatsuka M, Pyykko I, Farkkila M, Korhonen O, Starck JP: Blood pressure, flow, and peripheral resistance of digital arteries in vibration syndrome. *Br J Industr Med* 40:434, 1983.

Futatsuka M, Yasutake N, Sakurai T, Matsumoto T: Comparative study of vibration disease among operators of vibratory tools by factor analysis. *Br J Industr Med* 42:260, 1985a.

Futatsuka M, Ueno T, Sakurai T: Followup study of vibration induced white finger in chain saw operators. *Br J Industr Med* 42:267, 1985b.

Gurdjian ES, Walker LW: Traumatic vasospastic disease of the hand (white fingers). *JAMA* 129:668, 1945.

Hack M, Boillat M-A, Schweizer C, Lob M: Assessment of vibration induced white finger: reliability and validity of two tests. *Br J Industr Med* 43:284, 1986.

Hashimoto K, Craig RS: Acrosclerosis associated with vibration: an electron microscopy study. *J Cutan Pathol* 7:373, 1980.

Hellstrom B, Andersen KL: Vibration injuries in Norwegian forest workers. *Br J Industr Med* 29:255, 1972.

Hellstrom B, Stenavald I, Halvorsrud JR, Vik T: Finger blood circulation in forest workers with Raynaud's phenomenon of occupational origin. *Int Z Angew Physiol* 29:18, 1970.

Hyvarinen J, Pyykko I, Sundberg S: Vibration frequencies and amplitudes in the aetiology of traumatic vasospastic disease. *Lancet* 1:791, 1973.

Iki M, Kurumatani N, Moriyama T: Vibration-induced white fingers and hearing loss. *Lancet* 2:282, 1983.

Iki M, Kurumatani N, Moriyama T, Satoh M, Matsura F, Arai T: Hearing loss and vibration-induced white finger. *Lancet* 1:453, 1987.

Juul C, Nielsen SL: Locally induced digital vasospasm detected by delayed rewarming in Raynaud's phenomenon of occupational origin. *Br J Industr Med* 38:87, 1981.

Mackiewicz Z, Piskorz A: Raynaud's phenomenon following long-term repeated action of great differences of temperature. *J Cardiovasc Surg* 18:151, 1977.

Marshall J, Poole EW, Reynard WA: Raynaud's phenomenon due to vibrating tools: neurological observations. *Lancet* 1:1151, 1954.

Matoba T, Kusumoto H, Mizuki Y, Kuwahara H, Inanga K, Takamatsu M: Clinical features and laboratory findings of vibration disease: a review of 300 cases. *Tohoku J Exp Med* 123:57, 1977.

Matoba T, Ogata M, Kuwahara H: Diltiazem and Raynaud's syndrome. *Ann Intern Med* 97:445, 1982.

Miyakita T, Miura H, Futatsuka M: An experimental study of the physiological effects of chain saw operation. *Br J Industr Med* 44:41, 1987.

Miyashita K, Shiomi S, Itoh N, Kasamatsu T, Iwata H: Epidemiological study of vibration syndrome in response to total hand-tool operating time. *Br J Industr Med* 40:92, 1983.

Okada F, Honma M, Ui M, Kiyota N: Plasma guanosine 3′,5′-monophosphate responses to the cold pressor test in patients with vibration disease. *Arch Environ Health* 38:144, 1983.

Okada A, Inaba R, Furuno T: Occurrence of intimal thickening of the peripheral arteries in response to local vibration. *Br J Industr Med* 44:470, 1987.

Olsen N: Diagnostic tests in Raynaud's phenomena in workers exposed to vibration: a comparative study. *Br J Industr Med* 45:426, 1988.

Olsen N, Nielsen SL: Diagnosis of Raynaud's phenomenon in quarrymen's traumatic vasospastic disease. *Scand J Work Environ Health* 5:249, 1979.

Olsen N, Nielsen SL: Vasoconstrictor response to cold in forestry workers: a prospective study. *Br J Industr Med* 45:39, 1988.

Olsen N, Nielsen SL, Voss P: Cold response of digital arteries in chain saw operators. *Br J Industr Med* 38:82, 1982.

Olsen N, Fjeldborg P, Brochner-Mortensen J: Sympathetic and local vasoconstrictor response to cold in vibration induced white finger. *Br J Industr Med* 42:272, 1985.

Olsen N, Petring OU: Vibration elicited vasoconstrictor reflex in Raynaud's phenomena. *Br J Industr Med* 45:415, 1988.

Reiss F: Raynaud-like phenomenon produced by a sewing machine. *Dermatologica* 139:154, 1969.

Ryan T, Salter D: The effects of vibration on skin blood flow. *Bibl Anat* 16:180, 1977.

Stewart AM, Goda DF: Vibration syndrome. *Br J Industr Med* 27:19, 1970.

Takeuchi T, Imanishi H: Histopathologic observations in finger biopsy from thirty patients with Raynaud's phenomenon of occupational origin. *J Kumamoto Med Soc* 58:56, 1984.

Theriault G, DeGuire L, Gingras S, Laroche G: Raynaud's phenomenon in forestry workers in Quebec. *Can Med Assoc J* 126:1404, 1982.

Welsh CL: The effect of vibration on skin blood flow. *Br J Surg* 67:708, 1980.

Carpal Tunnel Syndrome

Aratari E, Regesta G, Rebora A: Carpal tunnel syndrome appearing with prominent skin symptoms. *Arch Dermatol* 120:517, 1984.

Bleeker ML, Bohlman M, Moreland R, Tipton A: Carpal tunnel syndrome: role of carpal canal size. *Neurology* 35:1599, 1985.

Dekel S, Papaioannou T, Rushworth G, Coates R: Idiopathic carpal tunnel syndrome caused by carpal stenosis. *Br Med J* 1:1297, 1980.

Ellis JM, Azuma J, Watanabe T, Folkers K, Lowell JR, Hurst GA, Ahn CH, Shuford EH, Ulrich RF: Survey and new data on treatment with pyridoxine of patients having a clinical syndrome including the carpal tunnel and other defects. *Res Commun Chem Pathol Pharmacol* 17:165, 1977.

Gelberman RH, Aronson D, Weisman MH: Carpal-tunnel syndrome. *J Bone Joint Surg* 62A:1181, 1980.

Gelberman RH, Hegenroeder PT, Hargens AR, Lundborg GN, Akeson WH: The carpal tunnel syndrome: a study of carpal canal pressures. *J Bone Joint Surg* 63A:380, 1981.

Hamlin E Jr, Lehman RA: Carpal tunnel syndrome. *N Engl J Med* 276:849, 1967.

Heller L, Ring H, Costeff H, Solzi P: Evaluation of Tinel's and Phalen's signs in diagnosis of the carpal tunnel syndrome. *Eur Neurol* 25:40, 1986.

Hoffman DE: Carpal tunnel syndrome. Importance of sensory nerve conduction studies in diagnosis. *JAMA* 233:983, 1975.

Layton KB: Acroparaesthesia in pregnancy and the carpal tunnel syndrome. *J Obstet Gynaecal* 65:823, 1958.

Linscheid RL, Peterson LFA, Juergens JL: Carpal-tunnel syndrome associated with vasospasm. *J Bone Joint Surg* 49A:1141, 1967.

Serra G, Migliore A, Tugnoli V: Raynaud's phenomenon and entrapment neuropathies. *Ann Neurol* 18:519, 1985.

Smith GP, Rudge PJ, Peters TJ: Biochemical studies of pyridoxal and pyridoxal phosphate status and therapeutic trial of pyroxidine in patients with carpal tunnel syndrome. *Ann Neurol* 15:104, 1984.

Stevens JC: The electrodiagnosis of carpal tunnel syndrome. *Muscle Nerve* 10:99, 1987.

Taylor N: Carpal tunnel syndrome. *Am J Phys Med* 50:192, 1971.

Walts AE, Goodman MD, Matorin PA: Amyloid, carpal tunnel syndrome, and chronic hemodialysis. *Am J Nephrol* 5:225, 1985.

Thoracic Outlet Syndromes

Adson AW: Surgical treatment for symptoms produced by cervical ribs and the scalenus anticus muscle. *Surg Gynecol Obstet* 85:687, 1947.

Adson AW, Coffey JR: Cervical rib: a method of anterior approach for relief of symptoms by division of the scalenus anticus. *Ann Surg* 85:839, 1927.

Banis JC Jr, Rich N, Whelan TJ Jr: Ischemia of the upper extremity due to noncardiac emboli. *Am J Surg* 134:131, 1977.

Beyer JA, Wright IS: The hyperabduction syndrome: with special reference to its relationship to Raynaud's syndrome. *Circulation* 4:161, 1951.

Conn J Jr: Thoracic outlet syndromes. *Surg Clin North Am* 54:155, 1974.

Lord JW, Rosati LM: Neurovascular compression syndromes of the upper extremity. *Ciba Clin Symp* 10:35, 1958.

Machleder HI, Moll F, Nuwer M, Jordan S: Somatosensory evoked potentials in the assessment of thoracic outlet compression syndrome. *J Vasc Surg* 6:177, 1987.

McGough EC, Pearce MB, Byrne JP: Management of thoracic outlet syndrome. *J Thorac Cardiovasc Surg* 77:169, 1979.

Roos DB: The place for scalenectomy and first-rib resection in thoracic outlet syndrome. *Surgery* 92:1077, 1982.

Roos DB: Thoracic outlet syndromes: update 1987. *Am J Surg* 154:568, 1987.

Rosati LM, Lord JW: *Neurovascular Compression Syndrome of the Shoulder Girdle.* New York: Grune & Stratton, 1961, p. 168.

Swinton NW, Hall RJ, Baugh JH, Blake HA: Unilateral Raynaud's phenomenon caused by cervical-first rib anomalies. *Am J Med* 48:404, 1970.

Telford ED, Mottershead S: Pressure at the cervico-brachial junction: an operative and anatomical study. *J Bone Joint Surg* [Br] 30:249, 1948.

Urschel HC Jr, Razzuk MA: Management of the thoracic-outlet syndrome. *N Engl J Med* 286:1140, 1972.

Urschel HC Jr, Paulson DL, McNamara JJ: Thoracic outlet syndrome. *Ann Thorac Surg* 6:1, 1968.

Wright IS: The neurovascular syndrome produced by hyperabduction of the arms: the immediate changes produced in 150 normal controls, and the effects on some persons of prolonged hyperabduction of the arms; as in sleeping, and in certain occupations. *Am Heart J* 29:1, 1945.

Hypothenar Hammer Syndrome

Benedict KT Jr, Chang W, McCready FJ: The hypothenar hammer syndrome. *Radiology* 111:57, 1974.

Conn J Jr, Bergan JJ, Bell JL: Hypothenar hammer syndrome: post-traumatic digital ischemia. *Surgery* 68:1122, 1970.

Herndon WA, Hershey SL, Lambdin CS: Thrombosis of the ulnar artery in the hand. *J Bone Joint Surg* 57-A:994, 1975.

Kleinert HE, Volianitis GJ: Thrombosis of the palmar arterial arch and its tributaries: etiology and newer concepts in treatment. *J Trauma* 5:447, 1965.

Little JM, Ferguson DA: The incidence of the hypothenar hammer syndrome. *Arch Surg* 105:684, 1972.

Millender LH, Nalebuff EA, Kasdon E: Aneurysms and thromboses of the ulnar artery in the hand. *Arch Surg* 105:686, 1972.

Mori KW, Bookstein JJ, Heeney DJ, Bardin JA, Donnelly KJ, Rhodes GA, Dilley RB, Warmath MA, Bernstein EF: Selective streptokinase infusion: clinical and laboratory correlates. *Radiology* 148:677, 1983.

Pineda CJ, Weisman MH, Bookstein JJ, Saltzstein SL: Hypothenar hammer syndrome: form of reversible Raynaud's phenomenon. *Am J Med* 79:561, 1985.

Vayssairat M, Priollet P, Capron L, Hagege A, Housset E: Does karate injure blood vessels of the hand. *Lancet* 2:529, 1984.

Vayssairat M, Debure C, Cormier J-M, Bruneval P, Laurian C, Juillet Y: Hypothenar hammer syndrome: seventeen cases with long-term follow-up. *J Vasc Surg* 5:538, 1987.

Obstructive Arterial Disease

Allen EV, Brown GE: Thrombo-angiitis obliterans: a clinical study of 200 cases. *Ann Intern Med* 1:535, 1928.

Goodman RM, Elian B, Mozes M, Deutsch V: Buerger's disease in Israel. *Am J Med* 39:601, 1965.

Hines EA Jr, Barker NW: Arteriosclerosis obliterans: a clinical and pathologic study. *Am J Med Sci* 200:717, 1940.

Hirai M, Shionoya S: Arterial obstruction of the upper limb in Buerger's disease: its incidence and primary lesion. *Br J Surg* 66:124, 1979.

Reflex Sympathetic Dystrophy

Drucker WR, Hubay CA, Holden WD, Bukovnic JA: Pathogenesis of post-traumatic sympathetic dystrophy. *Am J Surg* 97:454, 1959.

Polycythemia, Macroglobulins, Cryoproteinemias, Cold Agglutinins

Brown GE, Griffin HZ: Peripheral arterial disease in polycythemia vera. *Arch Intern Med* 46:705, 1930.

Carey RM, Wilson JL, Tamerin JA: Gangrene of feet and haemolytic anaemia associated with cold haemagglutinins in atypical pneumonia. *Harlem Hosp Bull* 1:25, 1948.

Diederichsen H, Clausen C, Lundborg CJ: Asymptomatic primary biliary cirrhosis associated with Raynaud's phenomenon, sclerodactyly and telangiectasia. *Dan Med Bull* 28:212, 1981.

Erf LA: A note of the stability of cold haemagglutinins. *Am J Clin Pathol* 15:210, 1945.

Hansen PF, Faber M: Raynaud's syndrome originating from reversible precipitation of protein. *Acta Med Scand* 129:81, 1947.

Hillestad LK: The peripheral circulation during exposure to cold in normals and in patients with the syndrome of high-titre cold haemagglutination. *Acta Med Scand* 164:211, 1959.

Imhof JW, Boars H, Verloop MC: Clinical haematologic aspects of macroglobulinaemia Waldenstrom. *Acta Med Scand* 163:349, 1959.

Invernizzi F, Galli M, Serino G, Monti G, Meroni PL, Granatieri C, Zanussi C: Secondary and essential cryoglobulinemias. *Acta Haematol* 70:73, 1983.

Jager BV: Cryofibrinogenemia. *N Engl J Med* 266:579, 1962.

Kramer DW, Perilstein PK: Case report of cold sensitivity with cold haemagglutinins. *Angiology* 2:283, 1951.

Marshall RJ, Shepherd JT, Thompson ID: Vascular responses in patients with high serum titres of cold agglutinins. *Clin Sci* 12:255, 1953.

McGrath MA, Penny R: Blood hyperviscosity in cryoglobulinemia: temperature sensitivity and correlation with reduced skin blood flow. *Aust J Exp Biol Med Sci* 56:127, 1978.

McLeod BC, Sassetti RJ: Plasmapheresis with return of cryoglobulin-depleted autologous plasma (cryoglobulinpheresis) in cryoglobulinemia. *Blood* 55:866, 1980.

Murray-Lyon IM, Thompson RPH, Ansel ID, Williams R: Scleroderma and primary biliary cirrhosis. *Br Med J* 3:258, 1970.

Nelson MG, Marshall RJ: The syndrome of high-titre cold haemagglutination. *Br Med J* 2:314, 1953.

Olesen H: The cold agglutinin syndrome. *Dan Med Bull* 14:138, 1967.

Reynolds TB, Denison EK, Frankl HD, Lieberman FL, Peters RL: Primary biliary cirrhosis with scleroderma, Raynaud's phenomenon and telangiectasia. *Am J Med* 50:302, 1971.

Ristow SC, Griner PF, Abraham GN, Shoulson I: Reversal of systemic manifestations of cryoglobulinemia. *Arch Intern Med* 136:467, 1976.

Ritzmann SE, Levin WC: Cryopathies: a review. *Arch Intern Med* 107:186, 1961.

Sherlock S, Scheuer PJ: The presentation and diagnosis of 100 patients with primary biliary cirrhosis. *N Engl J Med* 289:674, 1973.

Zinneman HH, Caperton E: Cryoglobulinemia in a patient with Sjögren's syndrome, and factors of cryoprecipitation. *J Lab Clin Med* 89:483, 1977.

Vinyl Chloride Disease

Falappa P, Magnaxita N, Bergamaschi A, Colavita N: Angiographic study of digital arteries in workers exposed to vinyl chloride. *Br J Industr Med* 39:169, 1982.

Harris DK, Adams WGF: Acro-osteolysis occurring in men engaged in the polymerization of vinyl chloride. *Br Med J* 3:712, 1967.

Johnston ENM: Vinyl chloride disease. *Br J Dermatol* 978:45, 1978.

Koischwitz VD, Marsteller HJ, Lackner K, Brecht G, Brecht Th: Veranderungen der Hand- und Fingerarterien bei der Vinylchoridkrankheit. *Fortschr Rontgenstr* 132:62, 1980.

Langauer-Lewowicka H: Nailfold capillary abnormalities in polyvinyl chloride production workers. *Int Arch Occup Environ Health* 51:337, 1983.

Langauer-Lewowicka H, Dudziak Z, Byczkowska Z, Marks J: Cryoglobulinemia in Raynaud's phenomenon due to vinyl chloride. *Int Arch Occup Environ Health* 36:197, 1976.

Maricq HR, Johnson MN, Whetstone CL, LeRoy EC: Capillary abnormalities in polyvinyl chloride production workers. *JAMA* 236:1368, 1976.

Markowitz SS, McDonald CJ, Fethiere W, Kerzner M: Occupational acroosteolysis. *Arch Dermatol* 106:219, 1972.

Ward AM, Udnoon S, Watkins J, Walker AE, Darke CS: Immunological mechanisms in the pathogenesis of vinyl chloride disease. *Br Med J* 1:936, 1976.

Neoplasms

Andrasch RH, Bardana EJ Jr, Porter JM, Pirofsky B: Digital ischemia and gangrene preceding renal neoplasm. *Arch Intern Med* 136:486, 1976.

Friedman SA, Bienenstock H, Richter IH: Malignancy and arteriopathy. *Angiology* 20:136, 1969.

Hawley PR, Johnston AW, Rankin JT: Association between digital ischaemia and malignant disease. *Br Med J* 3:208, 1967.

Palmer HM, Vedi KK: Digital ischemia and malignant disease. *Practitioner* 213:819, 1974.

Powell KR: Raynaud's phenomenon preceding acute lymphocytic leukemia. *J Pediatr* 82:539, 1973.

Taylor LM, Hauty MG, Edwards JM, Porter JM: Digital ischemia as a manifestation of malignancy. *Ann Surg* 206:62, 1987.

Wytock DH, Bartholomew LG, Sheps SG: Digital ischemia associated with small bowel malignancy. *Gastroenterology* 84:1025, 1983.

Hypothyroidism

Christensen NJ: Plasma noradrenaline and adrenaline in patients with thyrotoxicosis and myxedema. *Clin Sci Mol Med* 45:163, 1973.

Koehn MA, Schindler WJ, Stanton HG: Thyroid state and vascular reactivity in rats. *Proc Soc Exp Biol Med* 126:861, 1967.

Nielsen SL, Parving H-H, Hansen JEM: Myxoedema and Raynaud's phenomenon. *Acta Endocrinol* (Copenh) 101:32, 1982.

Peacock JH: The treatment of primary Raynaud's disease of the upper limb. *Lancet* 2:65, 1960.

Shagan BP, Friedman SA: Raynaud's phenomenon in hypothyroidism. *Angiology* 27:19, 1976.

Shagan BP, Friedman SA: Raynaud's phenomenon and thyroid deficiency. *Arch Intern Med* 140:832, 1980.

Stewart HJ, Evans WF: Peripheral blood flow in myxoedema. *Arch Intern Med* 69:808, 1942.

Hepatitis B Antigenemia

Cosgriff TM, Arnold WJ: Digital vasospasm and infarction associated with hepatitis B antigenemia. *JAMA* 235:1362, 1976.

Gocke DJ, Hsu K, Morgan C, Bombardieri S, Lockshin M, Christian CL: Association between polyarteritis and Australian antigen. *Lancet* 2:1149, 1970.

Kim WK, Koff RS: Coexistence of Raynaud's phenomenon and chronic active hepatitis with hepatitis B antigen. *Digestion* 11:152, 1974.

McMahon BJ, Bender TR, Templin DW, Maynard JE, Barrett DH, Berquist KR, Lum MKW, Mann CC: Vasculitis in Eskimos living in an area hyperendemic for hepatitis B. *JAMA* 244:2180, 1980.

Miscellaneous Etiologies

Bauer GM, Porter JM, Bardana EJ Jr, Wesche DH, Rosch J: Rapid onset of hand ischemia of unknown etiology. *Ann Surg* 186:184, 1977.

Engler HS, Freeman RA, Kanavage CB, Ogden LL, Moretz WH; Production of gangrenous extremities by intra-arterial injections. *Am Surg* 30:602, 1964.

Engler HS, Purvis JG, Kanavage CB, Ogden LL, Freeman RA, Moretz WH: Gangrenous extremities resulting from intra-arterial injections. *Arch Surg* 94:644, 1967.

Friedman SA, Novack S, Thomson GE: Arterial calcification and gangrene in uremia. *N Engl J Med* 280:1392, 1969.

Gipstein RM, Coburn JW, Adams DA, Lee DBN, Parsa KP, Sellers A, Suki WN, Massry SG: Calciphylaxis in man. *Arch Intern Med* 136:1273, 1976.

Hager DL, Wilson JN: Gangrene of hand following intra-arterial injection. *Arch Surg* 94:86, 1967.

Lappchen J, Ritz E, Koch A, Morl H, Bammer J, Ossenkop C: Raynaud-Phanomen bei dialysepatienten. *Dtsch Med Wochenschr* 102:521, 1977.

Nielsen SL, Lokkegaard H: Cold sensitivity and finger systolic blood pressure in hemodialysis patients. *Scand J Urol Nephrol* 15:319, 1981.

Rowell N: Digital ischemia due to vascular anomalies. *Br J Dermatol* 96:615, 1977.

Singer A: Raynaud's syndrome following self-administered intra-arterial barbiturate. *Mt Sinai J Med* 43:66, 1976.

Wakim KG, Jones JM: Influence of arteriovenous fistula on the distal circulation in the involved extremity. *Arch Phys Med Rehabil* 39:431, 1958.

7

Treatment

Most patients with Raynaud's phenomenon in the community setting are young women whose symptoms are not incapacitating. When they consult a physician, it is often for an explanation of their disease. This setting is especially so if there have been members in their families who have had surgical operations or amputations for other vascular diseases. After an adequate work-up to rule out secondary causes of vasospastic diseases (treatment of secondary Raynaud's phenomenon is covered in Chapter 6), the patients can be reassured that they have a benign and common disease that does not lead to loss of limbs. In approximately one of six patients there is a deterioration of their condition, although less than 1 percent require digital amputation. Serological abnormalities may not predict an adverse prognosis over the next decade in patients who present with Raynaud's phenomenon, no other symptoms, and a normal physical examination. Even the presence of sclerodactyly may not indicate a serious underlying disease. These facts are important for the physician to remember when counseling patients.

GENERAL MEASURES AND COUNSELING

Care of the Acral Parts

Patients are instructed that the hands and feet must be kept warm and dry; mittens are preferable to gloves, as the fingers can then share their heat. Patients must avoid touching cold objects such as cold drinks and frozen foods; attacks often occur in the frozen food section of supermarkets. Pressure on the digits plus cold seems to induce attacks more frequently than cold alone, as illustrated by the frequency of reports of attacks on grasping the steering wheel of automobiles on cold mornings. Of course, patients should be told to avoid stimuli they know produce attacks.

Dressing Appropriately

Reflex sympathetic vasoconstriction is explained so the patient realizes that the whole body must be kept warm to keep the fingers vasodilated. It is well established that the digital blood vessels dilate in an attempt to lose heat when the body is warm. Patients experience vasospastic attacks most often as the seasons change; therefore they must dress warmly, covering all parts of the body when spring or fall approaches. This point should be emphasized, as the mornings and evenings are often cool at such times. Although cold weather induces vasospastic attacks, patients frequently have attacks with sudden drops in environmental temperature even when the weather is warm. Air-conditioning in warm climates can be uncomfortable for the patient with Raynaud's phenomenon. For these reasons, moving to a warm climate is not always helpful. It is particularly important to recommend a warm hat that covers the forehead, as a considerable amount of body heat can be lost through this site. Also, the application of ice to the neck or other parts of the body (swimming in cool or cold water) induces vasoconstriction in warm digits.

Ancillary Aids

In the colder climates, some patients need more than warm clothing to keep the acral parts and body warm. Muffs and fur-lined boots may help. There are a variety of hand and foot warmers available, including chemical heat bags that last up to 6 hours and electrically heated gloves and socks operated by a battery pack worn on the belt (rechargeable and lasting 3 hours). Kempson and co-workers (1983) described electrically heated gloves for use by patients with Raynaud's phenomenon. They reported that 11 of 15 patients found the gloves helpful, but no formal study was done and the etiology of the phenomenon was not determined. There are also battery-operated hand warmers that are carried in pockets for use as needed. These devices are especially useful for patients who must work outside in cool or cold climates. Advice for obtaining these devices can be obtained from the Scleroderma Clubs in the United States or The Raynaud's Association in the United Kingdom. These two organizations are excellent resources from whom the more severely afflicted patients can obtain advice and moral support.

Tobacco Smoking

Although the relation to Raynaud's phenomenon is not established, tobacco smoking should be stopped because it is another sympathetic stimulus that vasoconstricts digital vessels. In one study of 69 male patients, however, no relation of tobacco smoking to the course of the primary disease could be determined (Hines and Christensen, 1945).

Care of the Skin

If the patients' hands are dry, a moisturizing ointment or cream should be applied frequently during the day to prevent cracking of the skin, which often leads to infections. When infections or ulcers occur, antibiotics should be chosen based on the results of culture and sensitivity studies, although an antistaphylococcal agent can be started immediately. Topical anesthetic ointments are helpful for controlling pain.

Swinging the Arms

One other simple method that may stop a vasospastic attack was described by McIntyre (1978). Two patients were able to stop attacks by swinging their arms in a counterclock movement as fast as possible for several seconds. The centrifugal force might increase the digital artery transmural pressure, acting to distend the vessels and relieve the spasm. In our experience, this maneuver works but only for some patients. Peterson and Vorhies (1983) were unable to find any objective or subjective improvement in patients with primary or secondary Raynaud's phenomenon; rewarming times after ice water immersion of the hand for 30 seconds were unchanged by the maneuver.

DRUG THERAPY

With an explanation of the disease and the institution of the above methods to avoid attacks, most patients require no other treatment. If the vasospastic attacks interfere with daily activities or work, or trophic changes appear, drug therapy should be instituted. However, it must be recognized that all agents used for this disease have side effects, and that the drug chosen may relieve symptoms but does not affect the underlying disease.

In treatment studies of small numbers of patients with Raynaud's phenomenon, there are positive and negative reports for most drugs. Even the same group of investigators have reported beneficial and no effect on the frequency and duration of vasospastic attacks for the same medication (Malamet et al., 1985; Rodeheffer et al., 1983). The etiology or the severity of the disease in the patients in each study may be part of the explanation. However, since only 50 to 70 percent of patients respond to medication, it is more likely that the benefit of therapy can only be determined by studying large groups of patients.

Calcium Entry Blockers

Calcium entry blockers have been studied extensively for the treatment of Raynaud's phenomenon. They selectively block the movement of calcium ions in the slow channel, which leads to reduced influx of calcium into the cells and thus decreased smooth muscle contractility. However, there is evidence that some of these agents have α-adrenoceptor blocking activity, a beneficial effect on red blood cell deformability, an antiaggregating action on platelets (Dale et al., 1983; Kiyomoto et al., 1983), and an ability to inhibit thromboxane A_2 synthesis by platelets. They have been shown to be particularly effective for inhibiting vascular responses evoked by α_2-adrenoceptor activity (Timmermans et al., 1983), and these receptors are predominantly activated during reflex sympathetic stimulation of body cooling (Coffman and Cohen, 1988).

Nifedipine

The calcium entry blockers differ in their cardiac and peripheral activity, with nifedipine having the most potent peripheral vasodilator action. Several placebo-controlled studies have showed that nifedipine in doses of 10 or 20 mg three times a day decreases the number and severity of vasospastic attacks in patients with Raynaud's phenomenon (Kahan et al., 1983b; Meyrick et al., 1987; Nilsson et al., 1987; Rodeheffer et al., 1983; Sarkozi et al., 1986; Sauza et al., 1984; Smith and McKendry, 1982; Winston et al., 1983). Patients with primary Raynaud's disease may receive the most benefit. Digital ulcers have been reported to heal in patients with scleroderma (Kahan et al., 1983a). Even children have benefited from treatment with nifedipine (Matussi et al., 1985). Up to two-thirds of patients are improved, but some show no response. A note of caution must be added, as a second study by one group did not find a decrease in the frequency of vasospastic attacks (Malamet et al., 1985) and another study found that the benefit seen during the first 5 weeks was less apparent during the fifth to tenth weeks of treatment (Sarkozi et al., 1986).

Objective tests such as rewarming time following ice water exposure of the hand, finger pulse wave amplitude, and finger systolic blood pressure at 15° and 30°C have not reflected the benefit seen with nifedipine, but Nilsson and co-workers (1984, 1987) did find increased finger systolic pressure at 5°, 10°, and 15°C in patients with primary or secondary Raynaud's phenomenon. In similar patients, Creager and co-workers (1984) showed that sublingual nifedipine decreased finger vascular resistance, but a significant increase in blood flow was not found owing to the decrease in systemic blood pressure (Fig. 7–1). Similar findings have been

Fig. 7–1. Control compared to peak response of fingertip vascular resistance following 10 mg nifedipine sublingually in ten patients with Raynaud's phenomenon (mean $\pm$ SEM). There was a significant decrease in vascular resistance with nifedipine. *Source:* Creager et al. (1984). Reprinted by permission of the C. V. Mosby Company.

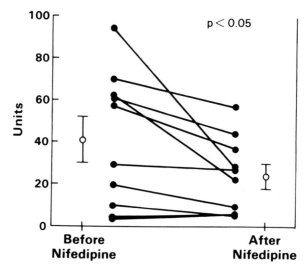

reported by two other groups who compared acute administration of nifedipine to placebo (Gush et al., 1987; Wise et al., 1987). Wollersheim and colleagues (1987) reported that 10 mg of nifedipine sublingually improved the finger skin temperature after hand cooling at 16°C for 5 minutes. However, in their chronic study of the oral drug in patients with primary or secondary Raynaud's phenomenon, no significant change occurred in skin temperature, laser–doppler skin blood flow measurements, or transcutaneous PO_2. Malamet and co-workers (1985) found that elevated levels of plasma β-thromboglobulin were lowered by nifedipine treatment but not by dazoxiben, a thromboxane A_2 inhibitor. Most of the patients had secondary Raynaud's phenomenon. This study indicates that in vivo activation of platelets was inhibited. The platelets could be activated in patients with Raynaud's phenomenon by vasoconstriction; it is less likely, but platelet breakdown could be of etiological importance.

Frequent side effects with nifedipine include headache (often transient), dizziness or lightheadedness, flushing, palpitations, and edema. Dyspepsia and pruritus may also occur. There is one report of treatment of the vasoconstriction of ergotism with nifedipine, but the vessels did not reopen for 2 days, which could reflect the natural course of the disease after ergot preparations are stopped (Kemerer et al., 1984).

Diltiazem

Three double-blind, placebo-controlled crossover studies (Kahan et al., 1985; Rhedda et al., 1985; Vayssairat et al., 1981) and one open study (Matoba et al., 1982) with diltiazem 30 to 120 mg three times a day have reported favorable effects in patients with primary Raynaud's disease or secondary Raynaud's phenomenon. Diltiazem significantly decreased the frequency, duration, or severity of vasospastic attacks in about two-thirds of patients. The open study was on patients with traumatic vasospastic disease; the rewarming time of hands immersed in 10°C water also was improved. Da Costa and co-workers (1987) reported the only adverse study; 12 patients with secondary Raynaud's phenomenon in a double-blind crossover study showed no decrease in the frequency of attacks or general improvement in their condition on 60 mg of diltiazem three times a day. There was also no improvement in finger blood flow (measured by impedance plethysmography) after 5 minutes of immersion of the hands at 5°C.

Side effects of diltiazem include headache, flushing, dizziness, nausea, and ankle edema.

Verapamil

Only one study has been reported on the use of verapamil (80 mg four times a day for 3 weeks) in patients with severe primary or secondary Raynaud's phenomenon (Kinney et al., 1982). Although 8 of 16 patients reported subjective improvement, their diaries of vasospastic attacks did not reflect it. No change occurred in finger systolic blood pressure, pulse wave form, total finger blood flow, or finger rewarming time after immersion in ice water for 20 seconds. Headaches and constipation occurred as side effects.

Nicardipine and Nisoldipine

Newer calcium channel blocking agents have also been studied. Intravenous nicardipine, 15 mg/hr, was compared to placebo, and it was found that it increased finger skin temperature and laser–doppler skin blood flow before and after cooling in normal subjects and in patients with primary Raynaud's disease but not in those with secondary Raynaud's phenomenon (van Heereveld et al., 1988). Rupp and co-workers (1987) administered nicardipine, 30 mg p.o. three times a day to 15 patients with secondary Raynaud's phenomenon and 12 patients with the primary disease in a parallel four week double-blind crossover study with placebo. In patients with primary Raynaud's disease, pain and frequency of attacks was improved by the drug, but only the number of attacks was reduced in the patients with the secondary phenomenon. No effect on finger blood flow (plethysmography) at rest or after a cold challenge was seen in either group. However, nicardipine, 30 mg p.o. three times a day, compared to placebo failed to reduce the number or severity of vasospastic attacks or to change objective tests in another study of patients with Raynaud's phenomenon (10 of 25 cases were primary). There was a reduction of plasma β-thromboglobulin and platelet factor 4 levels, suggesting that platelet activation is not of primary importance in initiating vasospastic attacks (Wigley et al., 1987).

Nisoldipine 20 mg daily was reported to decrease the frequency but not the severity of attacks in 19 patients with primary Raynaud's disease; no objective measurements were performed (Gjorup et al., 1986). In another study, 5 and 10 mg of nisoldipine were studied in a double-blind placebo controlled crossover trial in 36 patients with primary Raynaud's disease; no subjective improvement in symptoms or changes in resting finger blood flow (photoplethysmography), platelet aggregability, or red cell deformability were seen with the drug (Challenor et al., 1987). Since side effects occurred in 21 patients, the investigators considered the dose of the drug adequate.

Summary

Nifedipine and probably diltiazem have a place in the treatment of Raynaud's phenomenon. Nifedipine should be started at 10 mg three times a day and the dose increased if benefit does not occur and side effects allow. In our experience, approximately 50 percent of patients benefit. Nifedipine can also be used as a one-dose treatment at times of need, i.e., when the patient is to undergo severe cold exposure.

Sympatholytic Agents

Reserpine

Reserpine has been extensively studied for the treatment of Raynaud's phenomenon since 1958, when Burn and Rand reported that the accumulation of norepinephrine in arterial walls could be dispersed by reserpine and that nicotine and acetylcholine then lost their vasoconstrictor action. They suggested that the drug might be of benefit in Raynaud's phenomenon. Even low doses lead to the depletion of norepinephrine in dog femoral arteries (Porter and Reiney, 1975). Several uncontrolled clinical studies have shown that oral reserpine in doses of 0.25 to 1.00 mg per day benefits some patients with Raynaud's phenomenon (Coffman and

Cohen, 1971; Kontos and Wasserman, 1969; Peacock, 1960). There is no apparent method for predicting which patients will respond; patients with the primary disease and with secondary causes have benefited. Kontos and Wasserman (1969) showed that there was a decreased vasoconstrictor response in the hand (plethysmography) to intraarterial tyramine and to ice applied to the forehead following reserpine treatment, indicating that sympathetic nerves were affected. These authors also found norepinephrine undetectable in arterial or venous plasma after treatment. Coffman and Cohen (1971) demonstrated that reserpine increased the capillary blood flow in the fingertips measured by the disappearance rate of radioisotope in patients with primary or secondary Raynaud's phenomenon in both warm and cool environments (Figs. 7–2 and 7–3). This finding is important, as the disappearance rate of an isotope measures the nutritional blood flow of the digit.

Since the original favorable report of Abboud and co-workers (1967), studies concerning the use of intraarterial reserpine have produced variable results. However, parenteral forms of reserpine are no longer available in the United States. McFadyen and co-workers (1973) found no benefit when they compared it to pla-

Fig. 7–2. Capillary, total, and arteriovenous shunt flows in a 28.3°C room before and during reserpine treatment in a patient with Raynaud's phenomenon. Shunt flow is calculated by subtracting capillary flow from total flow. The capillary flow is similar before and during treatment; total and shunt flows are slightly larger during treatment. *Source:* Coffman and Cohen (1971).

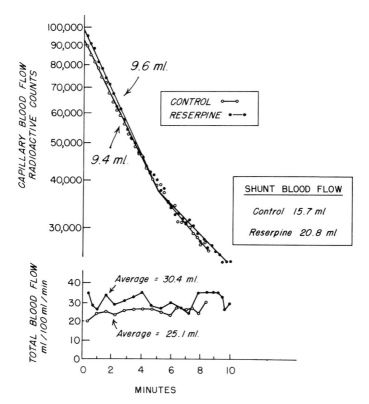

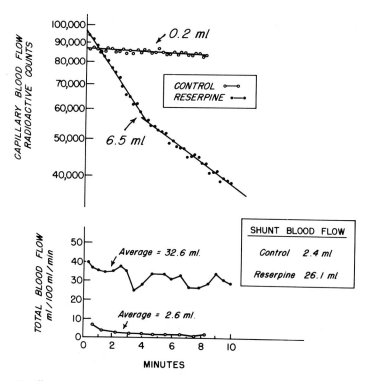

Fig. 7–3. Capillary, total, and arteriovenous shunt flows in a 20°C room before and during reserpine treatment for the same patient as shown in Figure 7–2. Shunt flow is calculated by subtracting capillary flow from total flow. During reserpine treatment the capillary flow increased from 0.2 to 6.5 ml; total and shunt flow also showed large increases. *Source:* Coffman and Cohen (1971).

cebo injections in patients with primary and secondary Raynaud's phenomenon at a dose of 1 mg. The number of vasospastic attacks, skin temperature, and discomfort index of patients given reserpine were unchanged compared to patients given placebo injections. Similarly, Surwit and co-workers (1983) found no benefit from bilateral brachial artery injections of a large dose of reserpine (1.5 mg in each arm) in similar patients. Compared to placebo there was no difference in frequency, duration, or severity of vasospastic attacks recorded by diary or in digital temperature response to a cool room challenge. Systemic reactions of increased stroke volume, bradycardia, and an increase in toe temperature did occur. Arneklo-Nobin and co-workers (1978) reported that 0.6 mg of intraarterial reserpine improved the level of pressure of digital artery closure and the clinical condition in six patients with primary Raynaud's disease, but the improvement lasted only 1 week. In patients with scleroderma and Raynaud's phenomenon, Nilsen and Jayson (1980) reported that the blood flow, as measured by the radioisotope technique, in the skinfold between two fingers increased after 1 mg of reserpine intraarterially for 1 to 3 weeks and as long as 5 months in one patient. The exaggerated reduction of skin blood flow with local cooling was also attenuated. Romeo and co-workers

(1970) also reported improvement in some patients for prolonged periods. Willerson and co-workers (1970) found that 7 of 13 patients with primary or secondary Raynaud's phenomenon improved with 0.6 mg of reserpine intraarterially and that esophageal motility normalized in two of five patients studied. In another study (Tindall et al., 1974), 1.0 to 1.5 mg of reserpine was injected intraarterially in 102 patients with Raynaud's phenomenon (50 with primary disease), and results were assessed subjectively. Sixty-six patients were said to have good or dramatic improvement, and 36 had little or no response. The beneficial effects often lasted 1 month.

Acevado and colleagues (1978) reported that 3 normal subjects and 15 patients with Raynaud's phenomenon (13 secondary cases) had an increase in digital blood flow (plethysmography) with 1.25 mg of intraarterial reserpine compared to that in the uninjected arm. The beneficial effect on cold sensitivity was said to last 1 to 5 weeks. Patients with only stellate ganglionectomy did not respond, whereas finger blood flow increased in the two patients with preganglionic sympathectomy.

Reserpine is of value in some patients with Raynaud's phenomenon of different etiologies. The dose should be 0.25 to 1.00 mg p.o. daily, starting with the small dose and increasing (or decreasing) the dose until there is relief of symptoms or production of nasal congestion or bradycardia to be sure an adequate dose is used. Side effects include bradycardia, postural hypotension, dyspepsia, fluid retention, lethargy, and depression. Reserpine should not be used in depressed patients or those with a history of depression. Gastrointestinal hemorrhage has been reported following the use of intraarterial reserpine. The advantages of reserpine are its low cost and once-a-day administration.

Guanethidine

Guanethidine interferes with the release of norepinephrine at the sympathetic neuroeffector junction. LeRoy and co-workers (1971) showed that guanethidine in doses of 30 to 50 mg p.o. daily for 4 to 6 weeks increased the capillary blood flow (xenon 133 disappearance rates) from the fingers in five patients with scleroderma during body cooling at 18°C. It is not mentioned if the frequency or severity of the patients' vasospastic attacks diminished. Strozzi and co-workers (1982) gave guanethidine at an average dose of 14.3 mg daily and compared it with methyldopa (704.3 mg daily) and debrisoquine (17.8 mg daily), another sympatholytic drug, in 21 patients with secondary Raynaud's phenomenon. The drugs were given for 6-week periods in a double-blind, crossover study. No drug was found to affect subjective complaints. The rate of skin temperature recovery after cold water immersion of the hand in 5°C water for 2 minutes improved with guanethidine and debrisoquine, but finger pulse waves were not significantly different. Other investigators have found guanethidine of value in the treatment of Raynaud's phenomenon in daily doses of 10 to 50 mg daily (Kontos and Wasserman, 1969).

Side effects include postural hypotension with lightheadedness or dizziness, diarrhea, and impotence. Guanethidine does not cross the blood-brain barrier and is therefore useful in patients who become depressed on reserpine. The agent should be started at 10 mg daily and the dose increased at weekly intervals until relief of symptoms or the development of side effects.

Methyldopa

The main action of methyldopa is evidently stimulation of central inhibitory α-adrenergic receptors, but methyldopa may also act as a false neurotransmitter, as it is metabolized to α-methylnorepinephrine. Varadi and Lawrence (1969) reported that approximately 75 percent of 42 patients with Raynaud's phenomenon of different etiologies benefited subjectively from methyldopa at a dose of 1 to 2 g daily. The beneficial effect was substantiated by an increased rate of rewarming of digits after exposure to cold as measured by skin temperatures. No controls were used in this study. As mentioned above, Strozzi and co-workers (1982) found no subjective or objective benefit in patients with Raynaud's phenomenon taking an average of 704.3 mg of methyldopa daily.

Side effects of methyldopa include edema, drowsiness, headache, diarrhea, dry mouth, postural hypotension, and nasal congestion. Rarely fever and hemolytic anemia occur. Methyldopa is not a first-line drug to be used in vasospastic disease but could be tried if other medications cannot be tolerated.

Prazosin

Prazosin is a specific α_1-adrenoceptor antagonist that has been recommended for the treatment of Raynaud's phenomenon since Waldo's (1979) report of the dramatic reversal of vasospasm and ulceration in a 60-year-old woman with primary Raynaud's disease. In a double-blind, placebo-controlled parallel study of 15 patients with primary Raynaud's disease, prazosin significantly reduced the frequency of vasospastic attacks, but finger systolic blood pressure was unchanged at 15° to 10°C (Nielsen et al., 1983). The highest tolerated doses, 2 to 8 mg daily, were used. However, the improvement tended to dissipate with prolonged treatment. Patients did not want to continue treatment because of the side effects.

In 20 patients with scleroderma and Raynaud's phenomenon, Surwit and co-workers (1982) found that the response of digital temperature to a 16°C environmental temperature was unchanged by prazosin, 1 mg three times a day, or by autogenic training for 4 weeks, although the two treatments together were successful. Symptomatic status was not mentioned in this study. Later, the same group reported that prazosin, 1 mg three times a day, decreased the frequency and somewhat the severity of vasospastic attacks compared to placebo in 19 patients with Raynaud's phenomenon due to scleroderma (Surwit et al., 1984). Unfortunately, the placebo patients had a similar good response in the crossover part of the study at 8 to 12 weeks, which could be explained only by milder environmental temperatures.

Russell and Lessard (1985) found no significant difference from placebo in the frequency of vasospastic attacks with prazosin, 2 mg twice a day, in 14 patients with Raynaud's phenomenon. A significant decrease in attacks was seen if the five patients with scleroderma were omitted from the analysis; those who benefited had other connective tissue diseases or the primary disease. In this study pulse volume of the digits did not change; finger systolic blood pressure during body cooling to 15°C did improve in the group only if patients with scleroderma were eliminated.

Wollersheim and co-workers (1986) compared prazosin, 1 mg three times a day, to placebo in a 2-week crossover study; there was moderate improvement in the frequency and duration of attacks in 24 patients with Raynaud's phenomenon.

Patients showed a preference for prazosin over placebo. Finger skin temperature and laser–doppler finger blood flow were significantly improved with the drug. Patients with primary Raynaud's disease and those with secondary Raynaud's phenomenon were benefited. The daily number of attacks decreased from 4.1 to 2.5, and two-thirds of the patients were said to have an overall good response.

Side effects with prazosin include nausea, headache, palpitations especially with exercise, dizziness, fatigue, edema, dyspnea, rash, and diarrhea. Most of these effects are dose-related, but syncope may occur with the first dose; a test dose of 1 mg should be given preferably at bedtime. A positive antinuclear antibody titer may develop.

Prazosin is evidently beneficial in some patients with Raynaud's phenomenon, although the evidence is conflicting regarding which patients may benefit. Moreover, the effect may dissipate with time. As with other sympatholytic agents, side effects may prevent its use.

Phenoxybenzamine

Phenoxybenzamine is a potent α-adrenoceptor blocking agent that has been recommended for the treatment of Raynaud's phenomenon. In an uncontrolled study, Moser and co-workers (1953) reported a decrease in the number, severity, and duration of vasospastic attacks with this drug, 20 to 50 mg three or four times a day, in 10 of 13 patients with primary or secondary Raynaud's phenomenon. In another uncontrolled study, Hillestad (1962) found that phenoxybenzamine did not decrease the frequency or duration of vasospastic attacks, increase hand blood flow (plethysmography), or hasten the rewarming of the hand after 15°C water immersion in four patients with primary Raynaud's disease. Seven patients with secondary Raynaud's phenomenon had a decrease in hand blood flow during drug treatment.

Only one placebo-controlled, crossover study has been performed with phenoxybenzamine, 10 to 20 mg daily, in 31 patients with primary and secondary Raynaud's phenomenon (Cleophas et al., 1984). The recovery of finger temperature 12 minutes after finger cooling at 16°C for 5 minutes was significantly improved at 4 and 8 weeks of drug therapy. However, it is difficult to be sure that patients had fewer or shorter vasospastic attacks from the methods of analysis of this study.

The side effects—postural hypotension, nasal congestion, palpitations, impotence, and gastrointestinal symptoms—often preclude use of phenoxybenzamine. Because of the high incidence of side effects, small doses (10 mg daily) are recommended initially with a gradual increase up to 30 mg four times a day.

Phentolamine

Phentolamine is a nonspecific α-adrenoceptor blocking agent. Only a parenteral preparation is currently available. Coffman and Cohen (1987) compared intraarterial phentolamine, nitroprusside, and nitroglycerin in normal subjects vasoconstricted by environmental cooling at 20°C. Phentolamine, 50 to 150 μg/min, was the most effective agent for increasing finger blood flow and was the only drug that consistently increased capillary flow (Fig. 7–4). Brecht and Hengstmann (1981) administered 0.05 to 10 mg of phentolamine as single brachial artery injections to five patients with Raynaud's phenomenon (probably secondary) with multiple dig-

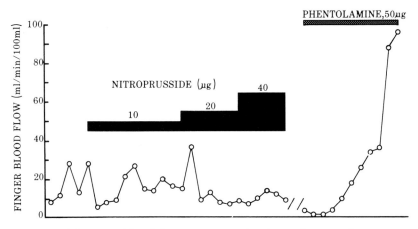

Fig. 7–4. Total fingertip blood flow in a normal subject during reflex sympathetic vasoconstriction induced by body cooling. No change in flow occurred with increasing doses of intraarterial nitroprusside. With intraarterial phentolamine there was a very large increase in flow. Flows are depicted at approximately 45-second intervals. *Source:* Coffman and Cohen (1987).

ital artery occlusions. Phentolamine produced a large increase in digital pulse volume amplitude and in forearm blood flow.

In fingers showing persistent, unrelenting vasospasm and ischemia, phentolamine given intraarterially is the agent of choice when the sympathetic nervous system is the cause. Systemic side effects are not usually seen.

Indoramin
Indoramin is an α-adrenoceptor blocking agent. Robson and co-workers (1978) studied this drug at a dose of 90 mg daily in 16 patients with secondary Raynaud's phenomenon. Seven patients who kept adequate diaries reported fewer vasospastic attacks per 2-week periods but not less discomfort. After an oral dose of the agent, patients showed an increase in finger blood flow for only 10 minutes and no change in digital temperature. Clement and co-workers (1986) administered indoramin 50 mg three times a day to 20 patients with primary Raynaud's disease in a double-blind, placebo-controlled, crossover study. Finger blood flow (plethysmography) increased significantly and the calculated vascular resistance decreased at 3 and 6 weeks. However, these authors found that the increase in blood flow was not significant after the fingers were immersed in 10° and 5°C water. It is doubtful that this drug is of value for vasospastic diseases.

Tolazoline
Parenteral or oral tolazoline increases skin blood flow in normal human subjects. It is an α-adrenoceptor blocking agent that also has a histamine-like effect. In vaso-constricted normal subjects, Coffman (1968) found that 100 mg of tolazoline given orally produced a small but significant increase in foot blood flow (Fig. 7–5). Moser and co-workers (1953) treated patients who had primary or secondary Raynaud's

phenomenon with tolazoline, 100 to 200 mg daily, but results were poor. Later, Prandoni and Moser (1954) treated nine patients who had Raynaud's phenomenon with a combination of oral and intraarterial tolazoline. Indolent digital ulcers healed after 3 to 5 weeks in five patients; the patients were subjectively better, but the oral preparation was not always effective. Coffman and Cohen (1971) reported that some patients who did not have an entirely acceptable response to reserpine benefited from the addition of tolazoline. No control studies have been performed. Adverse reactions include flushing, chills, scalp paresthesias, headache, palpitations, and gastrointestinal disturbances. The oral preparation of tolazoline has been withdrawn from the United States market.

Direct-Acting Agents

Nitroglycerin

Fox and Leslie (1948) and Lund (1948) reported beneficial effects of nitroglycerin ointment applied to the hands three times a day in several patients with severe Raynaud's phenomenon of questionable etiology. Nitroglycerin is a direct-acting vasodilator that has a greater action on veins than on the arterial circulation. However, Coffman and Cohen (1987) found that intraarterial nitroglycerin increased fingertip blood flow to a greater extent than did nitroprusside in vasoconstricted

Fig. 7-5. Total foot and calf blood flow and venous volumes measured by venous occlusion plethysmography in ten normal subjects in a 20°C room. Significant increases in foot blood flow occurred only with tolazoline (100 mg p.o.) and in calf blood flow with nylidrin (18 mg p.o.), tolazoline (100 mg p.o.), and isoxsuprine (40 mg p.o.). Venous volume showed a decrease with the same dose of nylidrin. *Source:* Coffman (1968).

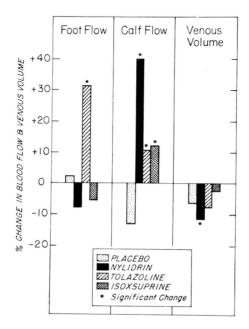

normal subjects. Kleckner and co-workers (1951) reported that 2% nitroglycerin in lanolin increased forearm blood flow and produced a variable increase in finger skin temperature in patients with Raynaud's phenomenon. The clinical response in their 25 patients was variable and temporary; the most consistent results occurred in patients with the primary disease. Peterson and Vorhies (1983) reported that only two of ten patients with primary or secondary Raynaud's phenomenon taking 0.4 mg of nitroglycerin sublingually showed improvement in the rewarming time of their digits after immersion in ice water for 30 seconds. Sovijarvi and co-workers (1984) could find no benefit from transdermal nitropaste plasters (12.5 mg once daily), when compared to placebo, in terms of the frequency or duration of vasospastic attacks or in the response of finger systolic blood pressure to graded cooling in eight patients with Raynaud's phenomenon (seven patients had the primary disease). However, Nahir and associates (1986) reported that a long acting, topically applied nitroglycerin patch (5 mg) decreased the frequency of attacks by 25% or greater, and the severity of attacks in a double-blind placebo controlled crossover study of 18 patients with primary or secondary Raynaud's phenomenon. Headaches and dizziness were a common problem, inducing 2 patients to withdraw from the study.

To avoid the problem of nitrite headaches, Franks (1982) treated 17 patients with secondary Raynaud's phenomenon for 6 weeks with 10 cm of 1% instead of 2% nitroglycerin ointment three times a day and compared the response to that with lanolin placebo. Patients on nitroglycerin had fewer and less severe attacks, and their ulcers healed better. All of these patients were already on maximally tolerated doses of sympatholytic agents. Fischer and co-workers (1985) did find a significant increase in finger blood flow in 22 patients with Raynaud's phenomenon, mostly primary in etiology, applying 800 mg of 2% nitroglycerin ointment. Systolic blood pressure and cardiac output decreased, and heart rate increased. Placebo ointment produced no changes. In an acute study, Coppock and colleagues (1986) applied five grams of 1% glyceryl trinitrate ointment to one hand and placebo ointment to the opposite hand of 17 patients with primary or secondary Raynaud's phenomenon. Although there was no change in finger systolic blood pressure at a local temperature of 30°C, there was a significant increase at 15°C in the drug treated extremity. This response suggested the effect of the drug was mediated locally. Contrary to the study of Kleckner and co-workers (1951), improvement was only seen in the patients with Raynaud's phenomenon secondary to an underlying connective tissue disease.

In all of the above studies, headache has been a main deterrent to using nitroglycerin ointment. Postural hypotension and paresthesias may also occur.

Although the study by Franks (1982) is impressive, our experience with the use of nitroglycerin ointment does not allow us to recommend its use. We have not seen benefit when it is used alone or in combination with other therapies. Contrary to the experience in patients with angina pectoris, patients with Raynaud's phenomenon often continue to have headaches.

Niacin and Derivatives

Niacin (nicotinic acid) and its derivatives cause flushing of the face and conjunctival injection; they produce more vasodilation of the blood vessels of the ears, face, and neck than of the extremities (Spies et al., 1938). In normal man, intravenous niacin may increase hand and forearm blood flow with only a slight increase in leg flow (Abramson et al., 1940). Holti (1978) reported that tetranicotinyl fructose in large doses produced a significant increase in skin temperature during a cold stimulus in patients with primary and secondary Raynaud's phenomenon. This drug is a fructose ester of nicotinic acid that releases nicotinic acid slowly in the small intestine so that a maximum effect occurs in about 4 hours. The side effect of flushing limited its use. Antcliff and associates (1974) showed that an acute dose of 250 mg of this agent increased finger blood flow (plethysmography) and reactive hyperemia in normals and patients with primary or secondary Raynaud's phenomenon, although the change was not large. It also prevented experimentally induced vasospastic attacks in five patients. Systemic blood pressure fell significantly, but flushing was the only side effect with this single dose. Arnot and co-workers (1978) administered the same drug at a dose of 500 mg three times a day for 2 weeks in a double-blind crossover study involving 12 patients with primary Raynaud's disease. No increase in finger blood flow was found by the xenon 133 disappearance rate technique; Arnot et al. mentioned, however, that six of seven patients had symptomatic relief.

Matoba and co-workers (1977) administered 200 mg of dl-α-tocopheryl nicotinate or placebo three times a day in a double-blind study of 60 patients with vibration-induced vasospastic disease. Patients were improved subjectively, and skin temperature recovery time after 10°C water immersion of a hand for 10 minutes was the only objective test that significantly improved.

Three studies have been performed with inositol nicotinate, but unfortunately none was suitably controlled. Holti (1979), after finding no effect of the drug in 2 weeks in a previous study, gave the drug for 12 weeks to 30 patients with primary or secondary Raynaud's phenomenon. Subjective improvement and an increased time to produce Raynaud's phenomenon was reported late in the study, but the weather had become warmer.

In an open trial, Aylward (1979) treated 20 patients with primary disease for 9 months with 3 to 4 g of inositol nicotinate daily. Patients were subjectively better, but there were no significant increases in hand blood flow or directly measured digital artery blood pressures. Digital artery blood velocity rate measured by a doppler technique did show an increase, but it is not a true indication of blood flow. Ring and co-workers (1981) used the same dose in 20 patients with the primary disease. They found a progressive improvement by thermography of the hands that was not significant until 36 weeks, and the skin temperature did not change after a cold stimulus in 15 patients tested. Patients reported a decrease in duration of attacks, coldness, pain, and numbness; frequency of attacks was not mentioned.

It is doubtful that these preparations are useful for treating vasospastic disease. The side effects—flushing, headache, and pruritus—are worse than the benefits reported.

Papaverine

Papaverine and its analogues dilate peripheral arteries in animals and man by a direct action on blood vessels. Even parenteral administration may produce only small increases in blood flow (Allen and Crisler, 1937; Littauer and Wright, 1939).

In Raynaud's syndrome of unstated etiology, Abramson and co-workers (1941) found little change in hand or foot flow with 30 mg of papaverine intravenously, whereas Mulinos and colleagues (1939) reported an increase in hand flow and skin temperature with papaverine, 60 to 120 mg i.v. three times a week. The large doses caused a depressed sensorium, facial flushing, perspiration, and increased respiratory and pulse rates. Controlled studies have not been performed.

Side effects of papaverine include flushing, malaise, gastrointestinal symptoms, and headache; hepatotoxicity has also been reported. Papaverine cannot be recommended for treatment of Raynaud's phenomenon.

Isoxsuprine

Because the chemical structure of isoxsuprine is similar to those of other β-adrenoceptor-stimulating drugs, its mode of action was assumed to be the same. However, it must have a direct relaxant effect on vascular smooth muscle, as β-adrenoceptor blocking drugs do not inhibit its action. In animal and human studies, isoxsuprine increases muscle blood flow, but skin blood flow is usually not affected.

In vasoconstricted normal subjects, Coffman (1968) found no change in foot blood flow after 40 mg of isoxsuprine was administered orally (Fig. 7–5). Wesseling and colleagues (1981) compared oral and sublingual isoxsuprine, at a dose of 20 mg, with placebo in a double-blind crossover study of seven patients with primary Raynaud's disease. By skin thermography, finger pulse waves, and skin temperature after cooling, the sublingual form was found to be superior to placebo or oral drug. No studies of subjective or objective improvement with the oral drug have been reported.

Isoxsuprine may cause palpitations, flushing, and postural hypotension. Because it does not increase skin blood flow, isoxsuprine cannot be recommended for the treatment of vasospastic diseases.

Griseofulvin

The antifungal agent griseofulvin has been shown to increase coronary blood flow and is thought to have a direct action in relaxing vascular smooth muscle. Sporadic case reports claimed improvement in patients with primary Raynaud's disease and with scleroderma (Creery et al., 1968; Giordano, 1967; Hasker, 1970). Charles and Carmick (1970) reported that six of seven patients with primary Raynaud's disease were subjectively better with 500 to 1000 mg of griseofulvin a day, but no placebo control was used in this study. During drug therapy there was also a more rapid skin temperature recovery after a 1-minute immersion of a digit in ice water. Sabri and co-workers (1973), in a double-blind crossover study, found that patients with primary Raynaud's disease preferred griseofulvin to placebo.

Side effects with griseofulvin include diarrhea, headache, indigestion, and dizziness. There is little basis to recommend griseofulvin for the treatment of Raynaud's phenomenon without a well controlled study. Our experience with this drug has shown there to be no benefit.

Cyclandelate

Cyclandelate (trimethylcyclohexanol) acts directly to relax vascular smooth muscle. In animal experiments, it has about three times the spasmolytic activity of papaverine. Van Wijk (1953) reported the use of 300 to 1000 mg of cyclandelate daily in patients with peripheral vascular diseases and found the least satisfactory results in patients with vasospastic disease. Four of six patients reported some improvement. Gillhespy (1956) treated 29 primary Raynaud's disease patients with 100 mg of this drug three times a day. Thirteen patients had a good response, eight a fair response, and eight no benefit. He considered that younger women with primary Raynaud's disease responded better than older patients. No controlled studies have been performed.

Side effects include nausea, heartburn, constipation, palpitations, headache, dizziness, and drowsiness. There is no evidence to support recommending this drug for vasospastic diseases.

Hydralazine
Hydralazine is a direct-acting vasodilator drug. Its use in patients with Raynaud's phenomenon has been reported as beneficial (Russell et al., 1985). Doses have ranged from 40 to 50 mg daily. No formal study has been reported.

Eicosanoid and Antiplatelet Agents

Dazoxiben
Dazoxiben is an inhibitor of thromboxane synthetase and also causes increased production of prostacyclin. Thromboxane A_2 is a potent vasoconstrictor and platelet aggregant. Therefore this imidazole derivative has been tested in patients with Raynaud's phenomenon, as it would block vasoconstriction of thromboxane A_2 in addition to inducing vasodilation from prostacyclin. Four studies (Coffman and Rasmussen, 1984; Ettinger et al., 1984; Jones and Hawkey, 1983; Luderer et al., 1984), which were double-blind and placebo-controlled, produced no benefit in patients with primary or secondary Raynaud's phenomenon at a dose of 100 mg four times a day. There was a small but significant decrease in the frequency of attacks and an increase in attack-free days in patients with primary Raynaud's disease on dazoxiben compared to placebo (Fig. 7–6) (Coffman and Rasmussen, 1984). Skin temperature, finger total and capillary blood flow, and forearm blood flow in warm or cool environments were measured in some of these studies and showed no change (Fig. 7–7). In one study (Tindall et al., 1985), the recovery time was faster after a challenge of cold air on the hand for 4 minutes, although finger blood flow (plethysmography) was unchanged at rest or during the cold challenge. A decrease in thromboxane B_2 and a rise in 6-oxo-$PGF_{1\alpha}$ during dazoxiben treatment was shown. In another double-blind, placebo-controlled study (Belch et al., 1983a), subjective evaluation by patients with primary or secondary Raynaud's phenomenon favored dazoxiben over placebo during the sixth week of treatment. Even in this study, hand temperature was not affected; in fact, hand temperature was decreased in the dazoxiben patients compared to that in the placebo group during the fourth week of treatment.

Dazoxiben cannot be recommended for treatment of Raynaud's phenomenon. The studies cited are pertinent in showing that these platelet products are probably not of etiological importance in primary or secondary Raynaud's phenomenon.

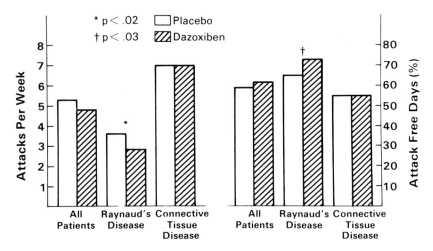

Fig. 7–6. Vasospastic attacks per week and percentage of attack-free days in 25 patients with Raynaud's phenomenon during placebo and dazoxiben (100 mg four times a day). When all subjects were considered, there were no significant differences between dazoxiben and placebo. Patients with primary Raynaud's disease showed a small but significant decrease in frequency of attacks and increase in attack-free days. *Source:* Coffman and Rasmussen (1984). Reprinted by permission of the C. V. Mosby Company.

Fig. 7–7. Finger blood flow measured by venous occlusion plethysmography, finger capillary flow by radioisotope disappearance rate, and digital systolic blood pressure in 25 patients with Raynaud's phenomenon during placebo and dazoxiben (100 mg four times a day). There were no significant differences in any parameter in either a warm (28.3°C) or a cool (20°C) environment. *Source:* Coffman and Rasmussen (1984).

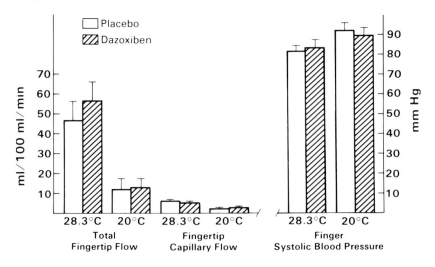

Prostaglandins

Prostaglandins that induce vasodilation and inhibit platelet aggregation have been studied for treatment of severe Raynaud's phenomenon. Both PGE_1 and epoprostenol (prostacyclin, PGI_2) have been used but must be given intravenously. Clifford and co-workers (1980) administered PGE_1 10 ng/kg/min for 72 hours to 26 patients with severe vasospastic disease. Patients reported less frequent and less severe vasospastic attacks, and digital ulcers healed in five of eight patients within 6 weeks. An increase in amplitude of finger pulsations and hand temperature occurred and lasted 6 weeks. There was no change in the rewarming time of the hands after immersion in 20°C water for 1 minute. The drug had to be given by a central intravenous line because of inflammation caused at peripheral sites.

Martin and co-workers (1980) administered PGE_1 6 to 10 ng/kg/min over 72 hours to 12 patients with scleroderma and compared it with saline infusions. The patients reported improvement of cold intolerance and reduced severity of vasospastic attacks with the drug; ten preferred PGE_1 to saline. Skin temperature rose an average of 2°C and was maintained for 2 weeks with the drug but not with saline. In two patients, finger ulcers healed. No serious side effects were reported. In a later study, these authors reported that PGE_1 increased capillary pressure, digital blood flow, and skin temperature (Martin et al., 1982).

Kyle and co-workers (1982) treated eight Raynaud's phenomenon patients with PGE_1 intravenously for 72 hours at a dosage of 6 to 10 ng/kg/min. Healing occurred in the five patients with ulcers, and all but one patient reported a decrease in the frequency of vasospastic attacks. Responses to a cold stress test improved and persisted for 2 to 6 weeks. Baron and co-workers (1982) also reported successful treatment of two patients with scleroderma and digital ulcers. Up to 50 ng of PGE_1/kg/min was given for 10 minutes every hour numerous times. Finger temperature increased and lasted 8 hours in one patient. Digital ulcers healed within 4 to 6 weeks, and digital pain was less. Allan and O'Reilly (1981) treated one patient with intravenous PGE_1 up to 10 ng/kg/min for 72 hours after sympathectomy and plasma exchange did not help. Hand and foot blood flow increased, as did tolerance to cool water. Objective measures had returned to pretreatment levels when measured at 31 days. The patient reported that there was no long-term improvement and no amelioration of vasospastic attacks.

In a multicenter study, intravenous PGE_1 for 72 hours was compared to placebo in 55 patients with Raynaud's phenomenon of primary etiology or secondary to scleroderma. PGE_1 showed no benefit over placebo in terms of frequency or severity of Raynaud's attacks, ulcer healing, skin temperature, or digital systolic pressure during cooling (Mohrland et al., 1985). Mizushima and co-workers (1987) studied the effect of PGE_1 incorporated into microspheres and given intravenously daily for 4 weeks. The lipo-PGE_1 is supposed to decrease inactivation of PGE_1 and irritation at the site of injection. Compared to placebo, there was no difference in Raynaud's attacks, but ulcers healed significantly better with lipo-PGE_1 in this study of 135 patients with severe vascular disease secondary to connective tissue diseases. Lucas and co-workers (1984) found an impaired deformability of erythrocytes in patients with severe Raynaud's syndrome (primary and secondary); intravenous infusions of PGE_1 for 72 hours did not improve erythrocyte filterability. Headache, flushing, diarrhea, postural hypotension, sweating, tachycardia, and a decrease in blood pressure may occur with PGE_1 infusions.

Dowd and co-workers (1982) administered prostacyclin (PGI_2) to 24 patients with Raynaud's phenomenon due to scleroderma at a dose of 2.5 to 10.0 ng/kg/min i.v. for 72 hours. Skin temperature was gauged by two methods in addition to the response to immersion of one hand in 20°C water for 1 minute. A large percentage of patients reported increased warmth of their hands and improved cold intolerance and pain in this uncontrolled study. The vasospastic attacks were alleviated for 4 to 28 weeks in 88 percent. Hand and finger temperature usually increased, but no difference was found in the response to cold stress after treatment. Hypotension, headache, facial flushing, abdominal colic, nausea, vomiting, and diarrhea were frequent side effects during the infusions. Pain at the angle of the jaw, sweating, dry mouth, and lassitude may also occur.

Belch and co-workers (1983b) administered prostacyclin 7.5 ng/kg/min for 3 weeks to seven patients with severe Raynaud's phenomenon of primary or secondary etiology; seven other patients received only the buffer. Prostacyclin reduced the frequency and duration of ischemic attacks and induced an increase in hand temperature. Clinical improvement was dissipated within 8 to 10 weeks, and hand temperature returned to baseline in 6 weeks. Other investigators (Rademaker et al., 1987) reported long-term benefit with an intravenous prostacyclin analogue in patients with Raynaud's phenomenon due to scleroderma. Without a control group of patients, such studies cannot be evaluated.

The same group (Belch and co-workers 1985) performed an interesting study with evening primrose oil in 21 patients with primary or secondary Raynaud's phenomenon. This naturally occurring seed oil contains γ-linoleic acid, the precursor of monoenoic prostaglandins. In a double-blind, parallel, placebo-controlled trial, the patients taking the 12 oil capsules daily had a decreased frequency and duration of vasospastic attacks compared to those ingesting placebo. The benefit did not reach significance until 6 to 8 weeks. No changes were seen in hand temperatures or digital systolic blood pressure during cold exposure. Significant changes in platelet function, PGI_2 metabolites, or thromboxane B_2 seen early in treatment did not persist during continued use of the oil capsules.

Much more investigation is needed before we will know if prostaglandins are of value in the treatment of Raynaud's phenomenon. The mechanism of the prolonged benefit reported in some studies is unknown; the inhibition of platelet aggregation disappears shortly after treatment (Dowd et al., 1982).

Van der Meer and associates (1987) studied the effect of acetylsalicylic acid, which inhibits platelet production of thromboxane A_2 and production of prostacyclin by blood vessels, together with dipyridamole, which induces a rise of the cyclic AMP content of platelets and plasma level of prostaglandin. For one week, 25 patients with primary or secondary Raynaud's phenomenon were given 80 mg of acetylsalicylic acid plus 75 mg four times a day of dipyridamole, acetylsalicylic acid plus placebo, or two placebos in a double-blind study. No significant changes in the symptoms of Raynaud's phenomenon or in the fingertip pulsation response to cooling or warming were found compared to placebo, despite demonstration of an inhibitory effect of the drugs on platelet function.

Serotonin Inhibition

Ketanserin

Ketanserin is a selective 5-HT$_2$ receptor antagonist that blocks the vasoconstriction and platelet aggregation induced by serotonin. It also possesses some α_1-adrenoceptor blocking activity. Stranden and colleagues (1982) demonstrated that intravenous ketanserin markedly increased digital pulse volume and finger temperature in nine patients with Raynaud's phenomenon, including six with the primary disease (Fig. 7–8). Saline injections were ineffective. Similar results were reported in another study during induction of vasospasm in a group of patients with Raynaud's phenomenon of diverse etiology (de le Fraille et al., 1986). Brouwer and co-workers (1987) also found a large increase in finger skin temperature and finger blood flow (plethysmography) with intravenous ketanserin in 11 patients with Raynaud's phenomenon. Since transcutaneous PO$_2$ did not change, they considered that nutritional blood flow was unaffected, although PO$_2$ may not always be an adequate indication of it. Seibold and Terregino (1986) found that intravenous ketanserin did not improve digital blood flow (plethysmography) if given before a cold challenge in four patients with primary Raynaud's disease, but it did produce vasodilatation if given during vasoconstriction. They concluded that serotonin may be involved in the maintenance of cold-induced vasospasm but not in its initiation. Longstaff and co-workers (1985) studied 23 patients with Raynaud's phenomenon (primary and secondary) in a double-blind placebo controlled study of ketanserin 40 mg twice a day for eight weeks. Ketanserin had no effect on doppler arterial

Fig. 7–8. Digital pulse volume (PVR), its first-order derivative (dPVR/dt), and skin temperature response to saline and ketanserin 10 mg i.v. No changes occur with saline, but large increases in pulse volume and skin temperature are seen with ketanserin. *Source:* Stranden et al., 1982. Reprinted by permission of the *British Medical Journal.*

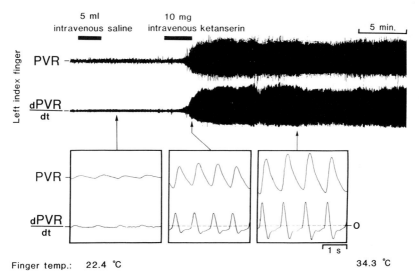

patency, laser-doppler digital blood flow, recovery time from a cold challenge, red cell deformability index, whole blood viscosity, β-thromboglobulin, platelet factor 4, or platelet aggregation responses. Symptoms were not reported.

In a double-blind, placebo-controlled crossover study (Roald and Seem, 1984), ten patients with Raynaud's phenomenon secondary to connective tissue disease were treated with ketanserin, 40 mg three times a day. Eight of the ten patients improved clinically, whereas none benefited from placebo. There was a decrease in number of vasospastic attacks per day and in the duration of the attacks. No significant increase in digital flow was measured by laser–doppler flowmetry, although red blood cells could be seen to flux earlier after the hand was cooled in water at 15°C for 2 minutes. Conversely, there was no difference in skin temperature recovery time after the cold exposure. Seibold and Jageneau (1984) reported similar results in an open study; 15 of 18 patients with scleroderma had moderate or marked relief of vasospastic attacks, but only 4 of 12 with Raynaud's phenomenon due to other etiologies benefited from ketanserin. They also thought that digital ulcer healing was facilitated and hand edema was less. An increase in maximal digital blood flow (plethysmography) was found at 38°C, and an improved blood flow was found during digital cooling in patients with scleroderma but not in patients with the primary disease or other connective tissue diseases. In a double-blind, parallel study of ketanserin (up to 120 mg daily), 5 of 7 patients with scleroderma showed improvement in qualitative finger blood flow studies and three had better healing, whereas none of the seven control patients showed improvement (Rovensky et al., 1985). Bounameaux and co-workers (1984), in a double-blind, placebo-controlled crossover study of ketanserin in eight patients with scleroderma found no benefit in terms of clinical improvement, frequency or duration of attacks, or finger systolic blood pressure at 30°, 15°, or 10°C. They used a smaller dose of ketanserin (80 mg daily). Also using the smaller dose of ketanserin, Kirch and colleagues (1987) compared it to nifedipine and placebo in a single-blind study of ten patients with Raynaud's phenomenon secondary to connective tissue diseases. Compared to placebo, neither drug produced a significant decrease in the frequency, duration, or severity of vasospastic attacks. Capillary velocity of red blood cells before or after a cold challenge was also unchanged, but both drugs increased skin temperature after warm water exposure.

In a double-blind, crossover study of ketanserin, 40 mg twice a day, and placebo in 41 patients with primary Raynaud's disease, van de Wal and colleagues (1985) reported no significant changes in frequency or duration of attacks, but the severity of attacks was decreased. There was also no change in skin temperature or digital systolic blood pressure in patients on ketanserin. Following the same patients in an open study, all parameters showed improvement over the initial data. Lagerkvist and Linderholm (1986) found that the same dose did not significantly influence skin temperature or finger systolic pressure during local cooling in arsenic workers or patients with primary or vibration-induced Raynaud's phenomenon. However, intravenous ketanserin 10 mg did increase the skin temperature and finger systolic pressure of cooled fingers in these patients. In another study of 9 patients with Raynaud's phenomenon due to the primary disease or scleroderma, the frequency and duration of attacks were unaffected and the finger temperature and recovery from a cold challenge was not changed by 40 mg three times a day of ketanserin (Brouwer et al., 1986). In a study of patients with traumatic vasospastic disease, oral ketanserin compared to placebo given during a double-blind crossover study did not significantly change the number of attacks, finger systolic pressure after cooling, or rewarming time after cooling (Larsen et al., 1986).

An international randomized, double-blind, parallel, placebo-controlled trial was performed with ketanserin, 40 mg three times a day, in 222 patients with primary or secondary Raynaud's phenomenon due to connective tissue diseases (Coffman, unpublished observations). There was a significant decrease in the frequency but not the duration or severity of attacks. The patients and their physicians considered they were improved by the drug. Patients with primary or secondary disease responded similarly. Finger blood flow (plethysmography) in warm and cool environments was not affected.

Side effects of ketanserin include dizziness, sedation, edema, dry mouth or eyes, anxiety, and scotomas. Ketanserin may be of value for treatment of primary and secondary Raynaud's phenomenon, but it must be taken three times a day and cannot be given with diuretics or antiarrhythmic agents due to prolongation of the Q-T interval. It is not yet available in the United States.

Angiotensin-Converting Enzyme Inhibition

Captopril

Captopril inhibits the production of angiotensin II from angiotensin I and also inhibits kininase II, allowing the vasodilator bradykinin to accumulate. Captopril was found to be especially effective for treatment of malignant hypertension associated with scleroderma.

Lopez-Ovejero and co-workers (1979) reported that two patients treated with large doses of captopril (600 mg daily) had excellent control of their blood pressure but also that their fingers became warm and digital ulcers healed within 5 to 6 weeks. They postulated that excess angiotensin may be important in the pathogenesis of the vasculitis seen with scleroderma. Miyazaki and colleagues (1982) treated one patient who had primary Raynaud's disease with captopril and reported remarkable improvement. However, they demonstrated that the acute vasodilator action of captopril on the fingers was blocked by serine proteinase inhibitors; infusions of angiotensin II antagonists had no effect on finger blood flow (photoplethysmography). They concluded that kinin accumulation caused by captopril was the main beneficial action. Trubestein and colleagues (1984) treated 20 patients who had primary or secondary Raynaud's phenomenon with captopril 25 mg three times a day and reported marked subjective improvement in 14 patients. It was an uncontrolled study. They measured an increase in finger systolic blood pressure, blood flow (plethysmography), and reactive hyperemia; finger blood flow increased significantly after cooling at 10°C for 10 minutes. In another uncontrolled study, captopril 25 mg three times a day was given to 63 patients with Raynaud's phenomenon for 3 months (Tosi et al., 1987). There was a significant decrease in the frequency and severity of vasospastic attacks in patients with primary Raynaud's disease but not in patients with scleroderma. There was also an improvement in finger blood flow (plethysmography) before and after a local cold challenge.

Captopril certainly has a place in the treatment of hypertension in scleroderma, but in our experience the peripheral vasospasm is often unchanged despite blood pressure control. It is also interesting that Wasner and co-workers (1978) reported remarkable regression of skin changes in three patients and improvement of Raynaud's phenomenon in two of these patients with scleroderma by controlling their blood pressure with hypertensive medications that did not include captopril.

BEHAVIORAL TREATMENT

Biofeedback and Conditioning

Many forms of behavioral therapies have been studied in an attempt to have normal subjects and patients raise the temperature of their fingers. Most are successful in some patients. They include autogenic training, which focuses on sensations of warmth and heaviness in the hands, muscle relaxation training with or without electromyographic feedback from the frontalis muscles, or any other method the patient wishes to use. Digital temperature feedback may be used with any of these techniques.

Lipkin and co-workers (1945), using a variety of methods, reported that mental suggestion improved several patients with primary or secondary Raynaud's phenomenon. They found no correlation between actual skin temperature and subjective sense of warmth. Surwit and co-workers (1978) found that autogenic training exercises and a combination of these exercises with skin temperature feedback produced the same significant improvement in the ability of patients with primary Raynaud's disease to maintain their digital temperature during a 17°C environmental cold challenge. A similar number of patients acted as controls and showed no improvement. Treated patients also had a significant reduction in the frequency of attacks per day.

The same group (Keefe et al., 1980) later compared autogenic training and general relaxation training, which included use of a sensitive temperature feedback device in the home. They found that the treatments were nonspecific and not related to skin temperature feedback. All treated patients showed an approximately 40 percent reduction in frequency of vasospastic attacks. These investigators also reevaluated 19 patients from their original study; all patients reported continued improvement 1 year after initial training, but their digital temperature response to the cold challenge had returned to pretreatment levels (Keefe et al., 1979). On the other hand, Surwit and co-workers (1982) treated 20 patients who had scleroderma and Raynaud's phenomenon with autogenic training plus placebo or prazosin. The patients were tested before and during treatment with a 42-minute 16°C environmental cold challenge. Only autogenic training plus prazosin raised the digital temperatures during the cold challenge. No other information is given concerning the clinical results in these patients.

Jacobson and co-workers (1979) treated 12 patients who had primary Raynaud's disease with 12 sessions of muscle-relaxing training; six patients also underwent auditory and digital temperature feedback. Both methods of treatment showed an increase in skin temperature. All patients reported their symptoms to be moderately to markedly improved at 1 month; seven patients were still improved at 2 years. The decrease in symptom severity did not correlate with the ability to raise digital temperature.

Freedman and co-workers (1981) reported ten patients with Raynaud's phenomenon who underwent 12 sessions of attempting to raise their finger temperature by any mental means; digital temperature feedback was used. There were no controls, but there was a dramatic decrease in the frequency of vasospastic attacks that was maintained for 1 year. Patients with the secondary phenomenon showed a better temperature increase during the sessions than patients with the primary disease. Finger temperature increases did not correlate with the decreased frequency of attacks. In a later study, the same group (Freedman et al., 1983) compared finger temperature feedback, finger temperature feedback during a cold stress, muscle relaxation with frontalis electromyographic feedback, and autogenic training. The first two methods increased finger temperature much more effectively. The patients who underwent sessions with finger temperature feedback during a cold stress had greater retention of voluntary vasodilation at follow-up in 1 year and a greater reduction in reported symptom frequency (92.5 percent).

Yocum and co-workers (1985) evaluated patients who had undergone biofeedback training at their institution after 1 year. The biofeedback consisted of muscle relaxation with electromyographic feedback followed by autosuggestions for relaxing and warming and home practice sessions of 20 minutes a day. On telephone contact, 57 percent of 18 patients reported subjective improvement and 44 percent of nine patients with digital ulcers noted benefit at 1 year. Four of seven patients could still elevate their finger temperatures 18 months after the training sessions, whereas all patients were able to do so during training. Similar to Freedman and colleagues, Yocum et al. found that patients with connective tissue diseases could raise their finger temperatures to higher levels than patients with the primary disease.

Jobe and co-workers (1982) used pavlovian conditioning to treat patients with primary Raynaud's disease. Eight patients and seven normal subjects, over a period of 3 weeks, underwent many sessions of immersing their hands in 43°C water while their bodies were exposed to 0°C temperatures. A second group of nine patients and seven normals acted as controls with no treatment. Digital temperatures during 0°C body cold exposure were measured at the end of the treatment period. The treated patients showed a significant increase in digital temperatures during the cold test and reacted similar to the normal subjects, whereas the untreated patients showed no change. Several subjects maintained this improvement up to 4 months. Patients also reported subjective benefit, and more than half of them had positive effects 9 to 12 months later. Similar results were reported in a later study (Jobe et al., 1985) when patients performed this conditioning program in their home environment. It is important to note that more severe cold stress was used in this study than in the biofeedback studies.

It may be concluded that biofeedback benefits some patients with Raynaud's phenomenon, including patients with connective tissue disease. It probably makes little difference what technique is used. If the pavlovian conditioning study is confirmed, it may be as good as or better than biofeedback; a more severe cold stimulus was counteracted, but the study did not detail clinical improvement compared to untreated patients. All these techniques do no harm to the patients and are worth a trial if the patient agrees. However, if biofeedback is used, the patient and physician must be willing to devote the extensive time involved.

PLASMAPHERESIS

Plasmapheresis, or plasma exchange, has been reported as a successful therapy for patients with severe Raynaud's phenomenon (Talpos et al., 1978). O'Reilly and coworkers (1979) compared plasmapheresis with placebo tablets or intermittent intravenous heparin therapy in 27 patients with Raynaud's phenomenon. At 6 months after plasma exchange, symptoms were still improved in five of eight patients, and more digital arteries were judged patent by doppler examination after 21° and 15°C water immersion in seven of eight patients. Digital ulcers healed in the three patients afflicted. There was no apparent difference in response between patients with primary or secondary disease. None of the patients on placebo or heparin showed any symptomatic improvement or increases in digital artery patency, but these modalities are not adequate controls for plasmapheresis, and digital artery patency determined by doppler examination is a questionable technique. In a later study, the same group (Zahavi et al., 1980) reported that plasmapheresis normalized the elevated β-thromboglobulin and platelet aggregation to adenosine diphosphate in patients with Raynaud's phenomenon. The effect lasted at least 3 months. Klinenberg and Wallace (1978) added a note of caution in that plasmapheresis did not improve Raynaud's phenomenon in a 50-year-old woman with rheumatoid arthritis or a 14-year-old girl with systemic lupus erythematosus.

Plasmapheresis may prove to have a place in the physicians' armamentarium of treatment for patients with severe Raynaud's phenomenon with digital ulcers unresponsive to other therapy. Weekly plasma exchanges of 2.0 to 2.5 liters for 4 weeks have been used in the above studies. It is an expensive procedure, and the risks associated with use of blood products are involved. Any improvement induced by the treatment occurs by an unknown mechanism. The importance of the technique may lie in determining the reason for the benefit reported by some patients, as it could lead to a new understanding of the pathophysiology and treatment of the disease. Van der Meulen and co-workers (1979) postulated that plasmapheresis may be beneficial because it removes the excess phagocytosed immune complexes they found in patients with secondary Raynaud's phenomenon.

MISCELLANEOUS TREATMENTS

Low-Molecular-Weight Dextran

Intermittent infusions of low-molecular-weight dextran have been used to increase digital circulation. Dextran 40 is a plasma expander that reduces red blood cell sludging, platelet adhesiveness, and blood viscosity. Usually 2 liters of 10% low-molecular-weight dextran in normal saline is infused over 48 hours. Holti (1965) reported that 10 of 12 patients with scleroderma benefited markedly from this treatment, with increased skin temperature, pain relief, and healing of ulcers. Two patients with the primary disease showed no change. In another study, 7 to 12 infusions of dextran were given to nine patients with scleroderma; most patients reported improved mobility of the fingers, less pain, and fewer vasospastic attacks, but there was no change in the cutaneous manifestations (Alani, 1970). Wong and co-workers (1974) demonstrated a small increase in forearm blood flow (plethysmography), capillary filtration coefficient, and $Na^{131}I$ disappearance rate in seven patients with scleroderma confined to the hands treated with dextran; beneficial effects in the fingers were reported in this uncontrolled study. Nordlind and colleagues (1981) used dextran to treat 12 patients with connective tissue diseases, and only five patients had increased capillary blood flow as measured by capillary microscopy. Of nine patients with ulcers, five had a beneficial response. Four of the 12 patients showed no improvement. In our experience, the hands and digits often become warm during the dextran infusions but quickly revert to their previous condition upon cessation of the dextran. If dextran infusions are used, patients must be monitored for fluid overload and pulmonary edema. Renal failure and anaphylactoid reactions are rare complications.

Hyperbaric Oxygen

Hyperbaric oxygen was used in one study to treat six patients with scleroderma and Raynaud's phenomenon (Copeman and Ashfield, 1967). Patients were exposed at two atmospheres of absolute oxygen for two daily sessions of 2 hours each for 10 to 14 days. Alleviation of the Raynaud's phenomenon was said to last longer than 1 month. Pain was relieved within 48 hours, and ulcers healed within 1 to 3 weeks in all of four patients.

β-Adrenoceptor Stimulation

Thune and Fyrand (1976) have treated patients with primary or secondary Raynaud's phenomenon using a β-adrenoceptor stimulating drug, terbutaline. Six of eight patients were better after a 5 mg dose three times a day. There was an increase in skin temperature and digital pulse wave amplitude in most patients, but two patients with scleroderma showed a decrease in both. Normal subjects showed a variable response to the drug, but control patients were not studied. Tremor and palpitations were reported side effects.

Fibrinolytic Enhancement

Jarrett and colleagues (1978) treated 20 patients who had Raynaud's phenomenon with an anabolic steroid, stanozolol, to enhance fibrinolytic activity. First, they showed that 24 patients with the primary disease and 26 patients with scleroderma had decreased blood fibrinolytic activity and increased fibrinogen. The drug was given in a 10 mg daily dose for 3 months followed by no treatment for 3 months, and then 3 months more of the drug in 20 patients with primary or secondary Raynaud's phenomenon due to scleroderma. They found an increase in hand blood flow (plethysmography) and an increase in palm and finger temperature during drug therapy; fibrinolytic activity was enhanced, and fibrinogen levels were decreased. Vasospastic attacks were less frequent, less severe, and of shorter duration in 80 percent of patients. The investigators postulated that reduced deposition of intravascular fibrin and an increased lysis rate of preexisting clot might explain the beneficial effect. Because of the side effects of tiredness, fluid retention, amenorrhea, acne, hirsutism, and the possibility of liver damage, they could recommend the therapy only as a last alternative. Their results have not been confirmed by others.

Transcutaneous Nerve Stimulation

Kaada (1982) studied the generalized vasodilation induced by local transcutaneous nerve stimulation in four patients with primary Raynaud's disease. He used low-frequency stimulation with constant square wave pulses of 0.2 msec duration for 30 to 45 minutes at 2 to 5 Hz and an intensity of 20 to 30 mA. A 7° to 10°C rise in skin temperature occurred that lasted from 4 hours to more than 8 hours. The patients used the stimulator at home, but only one patient continued to benefit. Three patients had migraine-like headaches after use of the stimulator. The mechanism of the induced vasodilation is unknown.

Dimethylsulfoxide

A double-blind multicenter controlled study compared normal saline with 2% and 70% topical dimethylsulfoxide for treatment of digital ulcers in 84 patients with scleroderma (Williams et al., 1985). No difference was found in any aspect of ulcer status or pain assessment with the two treatments. Significant skin toxicity occurred in more than 25 percent of patients using the strong solution.

Alcohol

Oral ingestion of alcohol produces vasodilation in the hands of normal subjects but decreases or has a variable effect on forearm blood flow (Graf and Strom, 1960). This effect is absent in sympathectomized or denervated limbs, so it is apparently mediated through the sympathetic nervous system (Fewings et al., 1966). A central action is favored, as muscle and skin flow are affected differently and intraarterial alcohol produces cutaneous and muscle vasoconstriction. Large amounts of whiskey, brandy, or other alcohol beverages must be consumed (90–150 ml) to relieve vasoconstriction, and thus there is the danger of intoxication. Vasko and Evans (1976) gave 10% ethanol 2 ml/kg/hr i.v. for 2 hours to eight patients with primary Raynaud's disease. Five of the eight patients developed pulsatile digital blood flow that was previously absent and a significant increase in dorsal hand temperature. No control studies have been performed, and because of side effects it is doubtful that alcohol has a role in vasodilator therapy.

Endocrine Hormones

Peacock (1960) considered that there was a relative hypopituitarism in patients with primary Raynaud's disease. If patients did not respond to reserpine, he added triiodothyroxine, 20 μg daily, as a second drug to increase the patients' heat production. Only 5 of 33 patients had no response to this regimen. Symptoms were alleviated in these five patients when intramuscular testosterone enanthate was given; methylandrostenediol 50 mg once or twice daily could be substituted for the more virilizing testosterone. There have been no further reports using thyroid preparations, but personal experience has not shown it to be beneficial in Raynaud's disease. The anabolic steroids have too many side effects to be considered for long-term use.

SYMPATHECTOMY

Extremities

Sympathectomy of the upper extremities has been used to ameliorate vasospastic attacks in patients with Raynaud's phenomenon. About 50 to 60 percent of patients have been benefited, with the best results in those with the primary disease (Baddeley, 1965; Birnstingl, 1967; Gifford et al., 1958; Hall and Hillestad, 1960; Kirtley et al., 1967; Laroche et al., 1976; Robertson and Smithwick, 1951; Tsur et al., 1973). Although immediate results are sometimes excellent, vasospastic attacks often recur within 6 months to 2 years (Felder et al., 1949; Johnston et al., 1965). A cure is uncommon. deTakats and Fowler (1963) considered that their 65 percent surgical success rate was due to the failure to recognize early cases of connective tissue disease. They believed the operation to be of no use for these diseases but valuable for Raynaud's phenomenon due to trauma, frostbite, emboli, thromboangiitis obliterans, atherosclerosis, or rheumatic arteritis, and for patients with "vasomotor hyperactivity." Various surgical procedures have been advocated, including postganglionic or preganglionic resection of the thoracic trunk and partial or complete removal of the stellate ganglion. Thoracic ganglia have been removed as low as T5. Although Robertson and Smithwick (1951) reported that preganglionic sympathectomy prevented return of sympathetic activity, most studies have not found a difference in the results of various procedures. Surgical approaches have been transaxillary, supraclavicular, or paraspinal with resection of the third rib; alternatively, an anterior thoracotomy was done. Transpleural and extrapleural exposures have been used. The extrapleural approach is associated with a lower complication rate.

Complications include pleural effusion, hemothorax, pneumothorax, atelectasis, neuralgia, wound hematomas and sepsis, and atrial fibrillation. Severe headache may occur with the paraspinal approach. After upper extremity denervation, Raynaud's phenomenon may be aggravated in the lower extremities. Horner's syndrome can be a bothersome result if the stellate ganglion is removed. Dryness of the skin, excess perspiration about the trunk and thighs, and a tendency to shivering in cool environments may occur.

With Raynaud's phenomenon of the toes, lumbar sympathectomy has been successful, with more than 80 percent of patients benefiting (Gifford et al., 1958; Janoff et al., 1985). The result is usually permanent, and cures are common.

Robertson and Smithwick (1951) found evidence of a return of vasoconstrictor activity to reflex cold stimulation after sympathectomy of the upper limbs in 65 percent of patients within 5 years and 80 percent within 5 years or more. The return of vasoconstrictor activity has been attributed to incomplete denervation, reinnervation (Simeone, 1963), or denervation hypersensitivity. Haxton (1947) and Simmons and Sheehan (1939) presented evidence for regeneration of sympathetic vasoconstrictor fibers following surgery. Haxton showed the return of sympathetic activity by demonstrating the presence of sweating using skin electrical conductivity measurements. The other group demonstrated the gradual return of sympathetic nerve activity by serial ulnar nerve blocks. Both groups concluded that local sensitivity of the blood vessels to cold also accounted for the failure of sympathectomy. Nielsen and co-workers (1980) found a local cold hypersensitivity in two patients after surgery. They postulated that it was probably due to degranulation of sympathetic vesicles and hypersensitivity to circulating catecholamines, as the venoarteriolar reflex was absent, indicating degeneration of vasoconstrictor fibers. However, it is still difficult to explain the remarkable results seen with lumbar sympathectomy on the basis of this theory. The failure of cervicothoracic sympathectomy is also used as evidence for Lewis's theory of a local digital artery abnormality in primary Raynaud's disease.

Local Surgery

Zook and co-workers (1978) treated six patients with ischemic fingers by resecting a portion of the thrombosed arteries. Four of the six patients had complete symptomatic relief, and two had definite improvement. In another patient, a vein graft to bypass the arterial obstruction was used and produced complete relief. It is postulated that resection of a portion of the artery produces sympathectomy of the vessel and therefore improves collateral circulation. Wilgis (1981) performed microvascular reconstruction of wrist or palmar arteries with vein grafts and reported that eight of ten patients had improvement of digital ischemia. He also performed 18 digital sympathectomies in ten patients by dividing terminal branches of the sympathetic nerves and stripping the adventitia from the common and proper digital arteries. Nine of the ten patients improved and had significant improvement in cold tolerance over 4 years.

Intravenous Sympathetic Blocks (Bier Block)

Local sympathetic nerve blockade can be produced by injecting sympatholytic agents intravenously (Hannington-Kiff, 1974). A needle is introduced into a peripheral vein in the hand or foot; the extremity is elevated, and the veins are emptied by compression with an elastic bandage. A blood pressure cuff on the proximal limb is inflated to suprasystolic pressure. Guanethidine (15–20 mg) or reserpine (0.5–1.0 mg) in 50 to 100 ml of normal saline is then injected into the vein, the larger amounts being used in the lower extremities. The arterial occlusion pressure is maintained for 15 to 20 minutes and then slowly released. Erikenson (1981) compared this technique with stellate ganglion blocks using 10 ml of 0.5% bupivacaine in 13 patients with Raynaud's phenomenon (probably the primary disease). The stellate blocks lasted less than 10 hours in four patients, whereas guanethidine (15 mg) Bier blocks lasted 3 days in nine patients as documented by skin temperature responses. Taylor and co-workers (1982) treated 14 patients who had Raynaud's phenomenon (probably secondary) and persistent digital ischemia with 0.5 to 1.0 mg reserpine by Bier block. Nine of 14 patients reported marked symptomatic relief for 7 to 14 days and had increased finger pulse waves. When using either guanethidine or reserpine, the patient must be carefully observed for postural hypotension after these procedures. We have used this technique only in patients with reflex sympathetic dystrophy, and the results have been variable. Parenteral preparations of reserpine and guanethidine are no longer available in the United States.

Cervicothoracic sympathectomy results are difficult to evaluate because probably only the most severely afflicted patients undergo surgery, and there are no controlled series. The success rate, however, is no better than conservative medical therapy in our experience. There is certainly no place for upper extremity sympathectomy in the treatment of Raynaud's phenomenon secondary to connective tissue disease, and it is of doubtful value for the primary disease. Lumbar sympathectomy successfully eliminates lower extremity digital vasospastic attacks but is seldom needed. We have seen worsening of upper extremity Raynaud's phenomenon following lumbar sympathectomy. The place of digital artery occlusion resection, vein bypass, or digital artery sympathectomy has yet to be determined. Intravenous sympathetic blockade is an alternative to stellate ganglion blockade or intraarterial administration of sympatholytic agents in an attempt to relieve persistent ischemia but has no place in the treatment of episodic attacks.

RECOMMENDATIONS FOR TREATMENT

Most patients with Raynaud's phenomenon, primary or secondary, should undergo a trial of conservative therapy before drug therapy is considered. Patients who have frequent vasospastic attacks that interfere with daily functioning, those with ulcers or gangrene, or those with painful attacks are the exceptions to this rule. The physician must explain the primary disease to the patient and the fact that it is a common, benign condition that does not lead to loss of limbs or digits. The patient should be instructed that not only the hands and feet but the whole body must be kept warm. The physiological reason for protecting the body from cold should be explained. Pressure plus cold on the digits should be avoided. Tobacco smoking must be stopped. Mittens are preferable to gloves. If the patient has the personality and time, conditioning sessions that immerse the hands in warm water while the body is exposed to cold temperatures, or biofeedback, is recommended, as this treatment is not associated with the side effects seen with medications.

If conservative therapy fails to give the patient adequate relief, drug treatment can be recommended. The sympatholytic agents and calcium-blocking drugs have yielded the best reults, with improvement occurring in about 50 percent of patients.

In our experience, patients who do not respond to one agent rarely are benefited by another type of medication. We have also not found that using two drugs that act by different mechanisms to produce vasodilatation yields more benefit than one agent.

Our current drug of choice is nifedipine, which is usually given in a dose of 10 mg three times a day, although doses as high as 30 mg three times a day have been used. If headaches occur, they usually dissipate within 2 to 3 days. Some patients do well with administration of nifedipine only before cold exposure, e.g., before driving to work in the morning or engaging in winter sports. Headaches often interfere with this regimen of intermittent dosage.

If side effects prevent the use of nifedipine, diltiazem 30 to 90 mg three times a day can be tried but is probably not as beneficial. One problem with the use of the calcium-blocking agents is the necessity of three-times-a-day administration. The sympathetic blocking drugs, reserpine or guanethidine, can be administered once daily, preferably at the hour of sleep. These agents are as effective as nifedipine in our experience but require careful dose titration. Patients should be started on the smallest dose, 0.125 mg of reserpine or 10 mg of guanethidine. The dose is then increased weekly until relief of symptoms or the occurrence of side effects. With reserpine, nasal congestion or bradycardia indicates that a therapeutic dose has been attained. With guanethidine, diarrhea occurs at the highest doses. Before each increase in dose, the patient should be checked for postural hypotension, which may occur with either drug. Usual doses of reserpine are 0.125 to 0.5 mg daily and guanethidine 10 to 50 mg daily. Guanethidine and not reserpine should be used in patients with a history of depression.

When these drugs fail to relieve the symptoms, we have had little success with other medications. In our experience, both prazosin and phenoxybenzamine have not been of long-term benefit, and the side effects with the latter drug are often intolerable. We cannot recommend nitroglycerin preparations. More experience with controlled studies is needed with intravenous prostaglandins or plasmapheresis before either can be recommended. Sympathectomy should be considered only for lower limb vasospastic disease.

REFERENCES

Abboud FM, Eckstein JW, Lawrence MS, Hoak JC: Preliminary observation on the use of intra-arterial reserpine in Raynaud's phenomenon. *Circulation* 36(suppl 2):49, 1967.

Abramson DI, Katzenstein KH, Senior FA: Effect of nicotinic acid on peripheral blood flow in man. *Am J Med Sci* 200:96, 1940.

Abramson DI, Zazella J, Schkloven N: The vasodilating action of various therapeutic procedures which are used in the treatment of peripheral vascular disease. *Am Heart J* 21:756, 1941.

Acevado A, Reginato AJ, Schnell AM: Effect of intra-arterial reserpine in patients suffering from Raynaud's phenomenon. *J Cardiovasc Surg* 19:77, 1978.

Alani MD: Treatment of scleroderma by Rheomacrodex. *Acta Dermatol* (Stockh) 50:137, 1970.

Allen EV, Crisler GR: Result of intra-arterial injection of vasodilating drugs on the circulation: observations on vasomotor gradient. *J Clin Invest* 16:649, 1937.

Allen JA, O'Reilly MJG: Treatment of severe Raynaud's phenomenon with prostaglandin E₁. *Ir J Med Sci* 150:190, 1981.

Antcliff AC, Bouhoutsos J, Martin P, Morris T: A plethysmographic study of the effect of tetranicotinoylfructose (Bradilan) on digital blood flow in primary and secondary Raynaud's phenomenon. *Angiology* 25:312, 1974.

Arneklo-Nobin BA, Nielsen SL, Eklov BO, Lassen NA: Reserpine treatment of Raynaud's disease. *Ann Surg* 187:12, 1978.

Arnot RS, Boroda C, Peacock JH: Pathophysiology of capillary circulation: Raynaud's disease. *Angiology* 29:48, 1978.

Aylward M: Hexopal in Raynaud's disease. *J Int Med Res* 7:484, 1979.

Baddeley RM: The place of upper dorsal sympathectomy in the treatment of primary Raynaud's disease. *Br J Surg* 52:426, 1965.

Baron M, Skrinskas G, Urowitz MB, Madras PN: Prostaglandin E₁ therapy for digital ulcers in scleroderma. *Can Med Assoc J* 126:42, 1982.

Belch JJF, Cormie J, Newman P, McLaren M, Barbenel J, Capell H, Lieberman P, Forbes CD, Prentice CRM: Dazoxiben, a thromboxane synthetase inhibitor, in the treatment of Raynaud's syndrome: a double-blind trial. *Br J Pharmacol* 15:1135, 1983a.

Belch JJF, Drury JK, Capell H, Forbes CD, Newman P, McKenzie F, Leiberman P, Prentice CRM: Intermittent epoprostenol (prostacyclin) infusion in patients with Raynaud's phenomenon. *Lancet* 1:313, 1983b.

Belch JJF, Shaw B, O'Dowd A, Saniabadi A, Lieberman P, Sturrock RD, Forbes CD: Evening primrose oil (Efamol) in the treatment of Raynaud's phenomenon: a double blind study. *Thromb Haemost* 54:490, 1985.

Birnstingl M: Results of sympathectomy in digital artery disease. *Br Med J* 2:601, 1967.

Bounameaux HM, Hellemans H, Verhaeghe R, Dequeker J: Ketanserin (5-HT₂-antagonist) in secondary Raynaud's phenomenon. *J Cardiovasc Pharmacol* 6:975, 1984.

Brecht T, Hengstmann JH. Therapeutic effects of intra-arterial phentolamine in "Raynaud's syndrome." *KLin Wochenschr* 59:397, 1981.

Brouwer RML, Wenting GJ, Visser W, Schalekamp MADH: Does serotonin receptor blockade have a therapeutic effect in Raynaud's phenomenon? *VASA* (Suppl) 18:64, 1987.

Burn JH, Rand MJ: Noradrenaline in artery walls and its dispersal by reserpine. *Br Med J* 1:903, 1958.

Challenor VF, Waller DG, Francis DA, Mani R, Roath S: Nisoldipine in primary Raynaud's phenomenon. *Eur J Clin Pharmacol* 33:27, 1987.

Charles CH, Carmick ES: Skin temperature changes in Raynaud's disease after griseofulvin. *Arch Dermatol* 101:331, 1970.

Clement DL, Duprey D, DePue N: Effect of indoramin on finger circulation in patients with Raynaud's disease. *J Cardiovasc Pharmacol* 8(suppl 2):S84, 1986.

Cleophas TJM, van Lier HJJ, Fennis JFM, van't Laar A: Treatment of Raynaud's syndrome with adrenergic alpha-blockade with or without beta-blockade. *Angiology* 35:29, 1984.

Clifford PC, Martin MFR, Sheddon EJ, Kirby JD, Baird RN, Dieppe PA: Treatment of vasospastic disease with prostaglandin E₁. *Br Med J* 281:1031, 1980.

Coffman JD: Effect of vasodilator drugs in vasoconstricted normal subjects. *J Clin Pharmacol* 8:302, 1968.

Coffman JD, Cohen AS: Total and capillary fingertip blood flow in Raynaud's phenomenon. *N Engl J Med* 285:259, 1971.

Coffman JD, Cohen RA: Intra-arterial vasodilator agents to reverse finger vasoconstriction. *Clin Pharmacol Ther* 41:574, 1987.

Coffman JD, Cohen RA: Role of alpha-adrenoceptor subtypes mediating sympathetic vasoconstriction in human digits. *Eur J Clin Invest* 18:309, 1988.

Coffman JD, Rasmussen HM: Effect of thromboxane synthetase inhibition in Raynaud's phenomenon. *Clin Pharmacol Ther* 36:369, 1984.

Copeman PWM, Ashfield R: Raynaud's phenomenon in scleroderma treated with hyperbaric oxygen. *Proc R Soc Med* 60:1268, 1967.

Coppock JS, Hardman JM, Bacon PA, Woods KL, Kendall MJ: Objective relief of vasospasm by glyceryl trinitrate in secondary Raynaud's phenomenon. *Postgrad Med J* 62:15, 1986.

Creager MA, Pariser KM, Winston EM, Rasmussen HM, Miller KB, Coffman JD: Nifedipine-induced fingertip vasodilation in patients with Raynaud's phenomenon. *Am Heart J* 108:370, 1984.

Creery RDG, Voyce MA, Preece AW, Evason AR: Raynaud's disease treated with griseofulvin. *Arch Dis Child* 43:344, 1968.

Da Costa JT, Gomes JAM, Santo JE, Queiros MV: Inefficacy of diltiazem in the treatment of Raynaud's phenomenon with associated connective tissue disease: a double blind placebo controlled study. *J Rheumatol* 14:858, 1987.

Dale J, Landmark KH, Myhre E: The effects of nifedipine, a calcium antagonist on platelet function. *Am Heart J* 105:103, 1983.

De la Faille HB, van Weelden H, Banga JD, van Kesteren RG: Cold-induced Raynaud's phenomenon ameliorated by intravenous administration of ketanserin: a double-blind cross-over study. *Arch Dermatol Res* 279:3, 1986.

DeTakats G, Fowler EF: Raynaud's phenomenon. *JAMA* 179:99, 1962.

Dowd PM, Martin MFR, Cooke ED, Bowcock SA, Jones R, Dieppe PA, Kirby JDT: Treatment of Raynaud's phenomenon by intravenous infusion of prostacyclin (PGI$_2$). *Br J Dermatol* 106:81, 1982.

Erikenson S: Duration of sympathetic blockade. *Anaesthesia* 36:768, 1981.

Ettinger WH, Wise RA, Schaffhauser D, Wigley FM: Controlled double blind trial of dazoxiben and nifedipine in the treatment of Raynaud's phenomenon. *Am J Med* 77:451, 1984.

Felder DA, Simeone FA, Linton RR, Welch CE: Evaluation of sympathetic neurectomy in Raynaud's disease. *Surgery* 26:1014, 1949.

Fewings JD, Hanna MJD, Walsh JA, Whelan RF: The effect of ethyl alcohol on the blood vessels of the hand and forearm in man. *Br J Pharmacol Chemother* 27:93, 1966.

Fischer M, Reinhold B, Falck H, Torok M, Alexander K: Topical nitroglycerin ointment in Raynaud's phenomenon. *Z Kardiol* 74:298, 1985.

Fox MJ, Leslie CL: Treatment of Raynaud's disease with nitroglycerin. *Wisc Med J* 47:855, 1948.

Franks AG Jr: Topical glyceryl trinitrate as adjunctive treatment in Raynaud's disease. *Lancet* 1:76, 1982.

Freedman RR, Lynn SJ, Ianni P, Hale PA: Biofeedback treatment of Raynaud's disease and phenomenon. *Biofeedback Self-Regul* 6:355, 1981.

Freedman RR, Ianni P, Wenig P: Behavioral treatment of Raynaud's disease. *J Consult Clin Psych* 51:539, 1983.

Gifford RW Jr, Hines EA Jr, Craig WM: Sympathectomy for Raynaud's phenomenon. *Circulation* 17:5, 1958.

Gillhespy RO: Treatment of peripheral vascular disease with "Cyclospasmol." *Angiology* 7:27, 1956.

Giordano M: Griseofulvin for scleroderma. *Lancet* 2:260, 1967.

Gjorup T, Hartling OJ, Kelbaek H, Nielsen SL: Controlled double blind trial of nisoldipine in the treatment of idiopathic Raynaud's phenomenon. *Eur J Clin Pharmacol* 31:387, 1986.

Graf K, Ström G: Effect of ethanol ingestion on arm blood flow in healthy young men at rest and during leg work. *Acta pharmacol et toxicol* 17:115, 1960.

Gush RJ, Taylor LJ, Jayson MIV: Acute effects of sublingual nifedipine in patients with Raynaud's phenomenon. *J Cardiovasc Pharmacol* 9:628, 1987.

Hall KV, Hillestad LK: Raynaud's phenomenon treated with sympathectomy. *Angiology* 11:186, 1960.

Hannington-Kiff JG: Intravenous regional sympathetic block with guanethidine. *Lancet* 1:1019, 1974.

Hasker WES: Griseofulvin in Raynaud's disease. *Lancet* 2:1136, 1970.

Haxton HA: Regeneration after sympathectomy and its effect on Raynaud's disease. *Br J Surg* 35:67, 1947.

Hillestad LK: Dibenzyline in vascular disease of the hands. *Angiology* 13:169, 1962.

Hines EA Jr, Christensen NA: Raynaud's disease among men. *JAMA* 129:1, 1945.

Holti G: The effect of intermittent low molecular dextran infusions upon the digital circulation in systemic sclerosis. *Br J Dermatol* 77:560, 1965.

Holti G: Experimentally controlled evaluation of vasoactive drugs in digital ischemia. *Angiology* 29:89, 1978.

Holti G: An experimentally controlled evaluation of the effect of inositol nicotinate upon the digital blood flow in patients with Raynaud's phenomenon. *J Int Med Res* 7:473, 1979.

Jacobson AM, Manschreck TC, Silverberg E: Behavioral treatment for Raynaud's disease: a comparative study with long-term followup. *Am J Psychiatry* 136:844, 1979.

Janoff KA, Phinney ES, Porter JM: Lumbar sympathectomy for lower extremity vasospasm. *Am J Surg* 150:147, 1985.

Jarrett PE, Morland M, Browse NL: Treatment of Raynaud's phenomenon by fibrinolytic enhancement. *Br Med J* 2:523, 1978.

Jobe JB, Sampson JB, Roberts DE, Beetham WP Jr: Induced vasodilation as treatment for Raynaud's disease. *Ann Intern Med* 97:706, 1982.

Jobe JB, Beetham WP, Roberts DE, Silver GR, Larsen RF, Hamlet MP, Sampson JB: Induced vasodilation as a home treatment for Raynaud's disease. *J Rheumatol* 12:953, 1985.

Johnston ENM, Summerly R, Birnstingl M: Prognosis in Raynaud's phenomenon after sympathectomy. *Br Med J* 1:962, 1965.

Jones EW, Hawkey CJ: A thromboxane synthetase inhibitor in Raynaud's phenomenon. *Prostaglandins Leukotrienes Med* 12:67, 1983.

Kaada B: Vasodilation induced by transcutaneous nerve stimulation in peripheral ischemia (Raynaud's phenomenon and diabetic neuropathy). *Eur Heart J* 3:303, 1982.

Kahan A, Amor B, Menkes CJ, Weber S: Nifedipine in digital ulceration in scleroderma. *Arthritis Rheum* 26:809, 1983a.

Kahan A, Weber S, Amor B, Menkes CJ, Saporta L, Hodara M, Guerin F, Degeorges M: Calcium entry blocking agents in digital vasospasm (Raynaud's phenomenon). *Eur Heart J* 4(suppl C):123, 1983b.

Kahan A, Amor B, Menkes CJ: A randomized double blind trial of diltiazem in the treatment of Raynaud's phenomenon. *Ann Rheum Dis* 44:30, 1985.

Keefe FJ, Surwit RS, Pilon RN: A one-year follow-up of Raynaud's patients treated with behavioral techniques. *J Behav Med* 2:385, 1979.

Keefe FJ, Surwit RS, Pilon RN: Biofeedback, autogenic training and progressive relaxation in the treatment of Raynaud's disease. *J Appl Behav Anal* 13:3, 1980.

Kemerer VF, Kagher FJ, Pais SO: Successful treatment of ergotism with nifedipine. *Am J Radiol* 143:333, 1984.

Kempson GE, Coggon D, Acheson ED: Electrically heated gloves for intermittent digital ischemia. *Br Med J* 286:83, 1983.

Kinney EL, Nicholas GG, Gallo J, Pontoriero C, Zelis R: The treatment of severe Raynaud's phenomenon with verapamil. *J Clin Pharmacol* 22:74, 1982.

Kirch W, Linder HR, Hutt HJ, Ohnhaus EE, Mahler F: Ketanserin versus nifedipine in secondary Raynaud's phenomenon. *Vasa* 16:77, 1987.

Kirtley JA, Riddell DH, Stoney WS, Wright JK: Cervicothoracic sympathectomy in neurovascular abnormalities of the upper extremities. *Ann Surg* 165:869, 1967.

Kiyomoto A, Sasaki Y, Odawara A, Morita T: Inhibition of platelet aggregation by diltiazem. *Circ Res* 52(suppl):115, 1983.

Kleckner MS Jr, Allen EV, Wakim KG: The effect of local application of glyceryl trinitrate (nitroglycerin) on Raynaud's disease and Raynaud's phenomenon. *Circulation* 3:681, 1951.

Klinenberg JR, Wallace D: Plasmapheresis in Raynaud's disease. *Lancet* 1:1310, 1978.

Kontos HA, Wasserman AJ: Effect of reserpine in Raynaud's phenomenon. *Circulation* 34:259, 1969.

Kyle MV, Parr G, Salisbury R, Thomas PP, Hazelman BL: PGE$_1$, vasospastic disease, and thermography. *Ann Rheum Dis* 41:310, 1982.

Lagerkvist BE, Linderholm H: Cold hands after exposure to arsenic or vibrating tools: effects of ketanserin on finger blood pressure and skin temperature. *Acta Pharmacol Toxicol* 58:327, 1986.

Laroche GP, Bernatz PE, Joyce JW, MacCarty CS: Chronic arterial insufficiency of the upper extremity. *Mayo Clin Proc* 51:180, 1976.

Larsen VH, Fabricius J, Nielsen G, Hanssen KS: Ketanserin in the treatment of traumatic vasospastic disease. *Br Med J* 293:650, 1986.

LeRoy EC, Downey JA, Cannon PJ: Skin capillary blood flow in scleroderma. *J Clin Invest* 50:930, 1971.

Lipkin M, McDevitt E, Schwartz S, Duryee AW: On the effects of suggestion in the treatment of vasospastic disorders of the extremities. *Psychosom Med* 7:152, 1945.

Littauer D, Wright IS: Papaverine hydrochloride: its questionable value as a vasodilating agent for use in the treatment of peripheral vascular disease. *Am Heart J* 17:325, 1939.

Longstaff J, Gush R, Williams EH, Jayson MIV: Effects of ketanserin on peripheral blood flow, haemorheology, and platelet function in patients with Raynaud's phenomenon. *J Cardiovasc Pharmacol* 7(suppl 7):S99, 1985.

Lopez-Ovejero JA, Soal SD, D'Angelo WA, Cheigh JS, Stenzel KH, Laragh JH: Reversal of vascular and renal crisis of scleroderma by oral angiotensin-converting enzyme blockade. *N Engl J Med* 300:1417, 1979.

Lucas GS, Simms MH, Caldwell NM, Alexander SJC, Stuart J: Haemorrheological effects of prostaglandin E$_1$ infusion in Raynaud's syndrome. *J Clin Pathol* 37:870, 1984.

Luderer JR, Nicholas GG, Meumyer MM, Riley DL, Vary JE, Garcia G, Schneck DW: Dazoxiben, a thromboxane synthetase inhibitor in Raynaud's phenomenon. *Clin Pharmacol Ther* 36:105, 1984.

Lund F: Percutaneous nitroglycerin treatment in cases of peripheral circulatory disorders, especially Raynaud's disease. *Acta Med Scand* 206:196, 1948.

Malamet R, Wise RA, Ettinger WH, Wigley FM: Nifedipine in the treatment of Raynaud's phenomenon. *Am J Med* 78:602, 1985.

Martin M, Dowd P, Ring F, Dieppe P, Kirby J: Prostaglandin E$_1$ (PGE$_1$) in the treatment of systemic sclerosis (ss). *Ann Rheum Dis* 39:194, 1980.

Martin MFR, Toske JE, Wright V: Microvascular changes produced by prostaglandin E$_1$. *Ann Rheum Dis* 41:309, 1982.

Matoba T, Kusumoto H, Mizuki Y, Yamada K: Comparative double-blind trial of dlα-tocopheryl nicotinate on vibration disease. *Tohoku J Exp Med* 123:67, 1977.

Matoba T, Ogata M, Kuwahara H: Diltiazem and Raynaud's syndrome. *Ann Intern Med* 97:455, 1982.

Matussi CM, Falcini F, Bartolozzi G, Volpi M: Nifedipine treatment of Raynaud's phenomenon in a paediatric age. *Int J Clin Pharm Res* 5:67, 1985.

McFadyen IJ, Housley E, MacPherson AIS: Intra-arterial reserpine administration in Raynaud's syndrome. *Arch Intern Med* 132:526, 1973.

McIntyre DR: A maneuver to reverse Raynaud's phenomenon of the finger. *JAMA* 240:2760, 1978.

Meyrick RH, Rademaker M, Grimes SM, MacKay A, Kovacs IB, Cook ED, Bowcock SM, Kirby JDT: Nifedipine in the treatment of Raynaud's phenomenon in patients with systemic sclerosis. *Br J Dermatol* 117:237, 1987.

Miyazaki S, Miura K, Kasai Y, Abe K, Yoshinaga K: Relief of digital vasospasm by treatment with captopril and its complete inhibition by serine proteinase inhibitors in Raynaud's phenomenon. *Br Med J* 284:310, 1982.

Mizushima Y, Shiokawa Y, Homma M, Kashiwazaki S, Ichikawa Y, Hasimoto H, Sakuma A: A multicenter double blind controlled study of lipo-PGE_1, PGE_1 incorporated in lipid microspheres, in peripheral vascular disease secondary to connective tissue disorders. *J Rheumatol* 14:97, 1987.

Mohrland JS, Porter JM, Smith EA, Belch JJF, Simms MH: A multicenter placebo-controlled, double-blind study of prostaglandin E_1 in Raynaud's syndrome. *Ann Rheum Dis* 44:754, 1985.

Moser M, Prandoni AG, Orbison JA, Mattingly TW: Clinical experience with sympathetic blocking agents in peripheral vascular disease. *Ann Intern Med* 38:1245, 1953.

Mulinos MG, Shulman I, Mufson I: On the treatment of Raynaud's disease with papaverine intravenously. *Am J Med Sci* 197:793, 1939.

Nahir AM, Schapira D, Scharf Y: Double-blind randomized trial of Nitroderm TTS® in the treatment of Raynaud's phenomenon. *Isr J Med Sci* 22:139, 1986.

Nielsen SL, Olsen N, Henriksen O: Cold hypersensitivity after sympathectomy for Raynaud's disease. *Scand J Thorac Cardiovasc Surg* 14:109, 1980.

Nielsen SL, Vithing K, Rasmussen K: Prazosin treatment of primary Raynaud's phenomenon. *Eur J Clin Pharmacol* 24:421, 1983.

Nilsen KH, Jayson MIV: Cutaneous microcirculation in systemic sclerosis and response to intra-arterial reserpine. *Br J Med* 1:1408, 1980.

Nilsson H, Jonasson T, Ringqvist I: Treatment of digital vasospastic disease with the calcium-entry blocker nifedipine. *Acta Med Scand* 215:135, 1984.

Nilsson H, Jonasson T, Leppert J, Ringqvist I: The effect of the calcium entry blocker nifedipine on cold-induced digital vasospasm. *Acta Med Scand* 221:53, 1987.

Nordlind K, Berglund B, Swanbeck G, Hedlin H: Low molecular weight dextran therapy for digital ischemia due to collagen vascular disease. *Dermatologica* 163:353, 1981.

O'Reilly MJG, Talpos G, Roberts VC, White JM, Cotton LT: Controlled trial of plasma exchange in treatment of Raynaud's syndrome. *Br Med J* 1:1113, 1979.

Peacock JH: The treatment of primary Raynaud's disease of the upper limb. *Lancet* 2:65, 1960.

Peterson LL, Vorhies C: Raynaud's syndrome. *Arch Dermatol* 119:396, 1983.

Porter JM, Reiney CG: Effect of low dose intra-arterial reserpine on vascular wall norepinephrine content. *Ann Surg* 182:50, 1975.

Prandoni AG, Moser M: Clinical Appraisal of intra-arterial Priscoline therapy in the management of peripheral arterial disease. *Circulation* 9:73, 1954.

Rademaker M, Thomas RHM, Provost G, Beacham JA, Cooke ED, Kirby JD: Prolonged increase in digital blood flow following Iloprost infusion in patients with systemic sclerosis. *Postgrad Med J* 63:617, 1987.

Rhedda A, McCans J, Willan AR, Ford PM: A double blind placebo controlled crossover randomized trial of diltiazem in Raynaud's phenomenon. *J Rheumatol* 12:724, 1985.

Ring EFJ, Ports LO, Bacon PA: Quantitative thermal imaging to assess inositol nicotinate treatment for Raynaud's syndrome. *J Int Med Res* 9:393, 1981.

Roald OK, Seem E: Treatment of Raynaud's phenomenon with ketanserin in patients with connective tissue disorders. *Br Med J* 289:577, 1984.

Robertson CW, Smithwick RH: The recurrence of vasoconstrictor activity after limb sympathectomy in Raynaud's disease and allied vasomotor states. *N Engl J Med* 245:317, 1951.

Robson P, Pearce V, Antcliff AC, Hamilton M: Double-blind trial of Indoramin in digital artery ischemia. *Br J Clin Pharmacol* 6:88, 1978.

Rodeheffer RJ, Rommer JA, Wigley F, Smith CR: Controlled double-blind trial of nifedipine in the treatment of Raynaud's phenomenon. *N Engl J Med* 308:880, 1983.

Romeo SG, Whalen RE, Tindall JP: Intra-arterial administration of reserpine. *Arch Intern Med* 125:825, 1970.

Rovensky LJ, Tauchmannova H, Zitnan D: Effect of ketanserin on Raynaud's phenomenon in progressive systemic sclerosis: a double-blind trial. *Drug Exp Clin Res* 11:659, 1985.

Rupp PAF, Mellinger S, Kohler J, Dorsey JK, Furst DE: Nicardipine for the treatment of Raynaud's phenomena: a double blind crossover trial of a new calcium entry blocker. *J Rheumatol* 14:745, 1987.

Russell IJ, Lessard JA: Prazosin treatment of Raynaud's phenomenon: a double blind single crossover study. *J Rheumatol* 12:94, 1985.

Russell IJ, Walsh RA: Selection of vasodilator therapy for severe Raynaud's phenomenon by sequential arterial infusions. *Ann Rheum Dis* 44:151, 1985.

Sabri S, Roberts VC, Higgins RF, Cotton LT, Williams DI: A double-blind clinical trial of griseofulvin in patients with Raynaud's phenomenon. *Postgrad Med J* 49:641, 1973.

Sarkozi J, Bookman AAM, Mahon W, Ramsay C, Detsky AS, Keystone EC: Nifedipine in the treatment of idiopathic Raynaud's syndrome. *J Rheumatol* 13:331, 1986.

Sauza J, Kraus A, Gonzalez-Amaro R, Alarcon-Segovia D: Effect of the calcium channel blocker nifedipine on Raynaud's phenomenon: a controlled double blind trial. *J Rheumatol* 11:362, 1984.

Seibold JR, Jageneau AHM: Treatment of Raynaud's phenomenon with ketanserin, a selective antagonist of the serotonin$_2$ (5-HT$_2$) receptor. *Arthritis Rheum* 27:139, 1984.

Seibold JR, Terregino CA: Selective antagonism of S$_2$-serotonergic receptors relieves but does not prevent cold induced vasoconstriction in primary Raynaud's phenomenon. *J Rheumatol* 13:337, 1986.

Simeone FA: Intravascular pressure, vascular tone, and sympathectomy. *Surgery* 53:1, 1963.

Simmons HT, Sheehan D: The causes of relapse following sympathectomy of the arm. *Br J Surg* 27:234, 1939.

Smith CD, McKendry RVR: Controlled trial of nifedipine in the treatment of Raynaud's phenomenon. *Lancet* 2:1299, 1982.

Sovijarvi ARA, Siitonen L, Anderson P: Transdermal nitroglycerin in the treatment of Raynaud's phenomenon: analysis of digital blood pressure changes after cold provocation. *Curr Ther Res* 35:832, 1984.

Spies TD, Bean WB, Stone RE: Treatment of classic pellagra: use of nicotinic acid, nicotinic acid amide, and sodium nicotinate, with special reference to the vasodilator action and the effect on mental symptoms. *JAMA* 111:584, 1938.

Stranden E, Roald OK, Krohg K: Treatment of Raynaud's phenomenon with the 5-HT$_2$-receptor antagonist ketanserin. *Br Med J* 285:1069, 1982.

Strozzi G, Cocco G, DeGregori D, Bulgarelli R, Padua A, Sfrisi C: Management of Raynaud's phenomenon with drugs affecting the sympathetic nervous system. *Curr Ther Res* 32:225, 1982.

Surwit RS, Pilon RN, Fenton CH: Behavioral treatment of Raynaud's disease. *J Behav Med* 1:323, 1978.

Surwit RS, Allen LM, Gilgor RS, Duvic M: The combined effect of prazosin and autogenic training on cold reactivity in Raynaud's phenomenon. *Biofeedback Self-Regul* 7:537, 1982.

Surwit RS, Gilgor RS, Duvic M, Allen LM, Neal JA: Intra-arterial reserpine for Raynaud's syndrome. *Arch Dermatol* 119:733, 1983.

Surwit RS, Gilgor RS, Allen LM, Duvic M: A double-blind study of prazosin in the treatment of Raynaud's phenomenon in scleroderma. *Arch Dermatol* 120:329, 1984.

Talpos G, Horrocks M, White JM, Cotton LT: Plasmapheresis in Raynaud's disease. *Lancet* 1:416, 1978.

Taylor LM Jr, Rivers SP, Keller FS, Baur GM, Porter JM: Treatment of finger ischemia with Bier block reserpine. *Surg Gynecol Obstet* 154:39, 1982.

Thune P, Fyrand O: Further observations on the therapy with a beta-stimulating agent in Raynaud's phenomenon. *Acta Chir Scand* 465(suppl):84, 1976.

Timmermans PB, van Meel JCA, van Zwieten PA: Calcium antagonists and alpha receptors. *Eur Heart J* 4(suppl C):11, 1983.

Tindall H, Tooke JE, Menys VC, Martin MFR, Davies JA: Effect of dazoxiben, a thromboxane synthetase inhibitor on skin blood flow following cold challenge in patients with Raynaud's phenomenon. *Eur J Clin Invest* 15:20, 1985.

Tindall JP, Whalen RF, Burton EE Jr: Medical uses of intra-arterial injections of reserpine. *Arch Dermatol* 110:233, 1974.

Tosi S, Marchesoni A, Messina K, Bellintani C, Sironi G, Faravelli C: Treatment of Raynaud's phenomenon with captopril. *Drugs Exp Clin Res* 13:37, 1987.

Trubestein G, Wigger E, Trubestein R, Ludwig M, Wilgalis M, Stumpe KO: Behandling des Raynaud-Syndroms mit Captopril. *Dtsch Med Wochenschr* 109:857, 1984.

Tsur N, Adar R, Bechor I, Bogokowsky H, Mozes M: Upper thoracic sympathectomy. *Is J Med Sci* 9:53, 1973.

Van der Meer J, Wouda AA, Kallenberg CGM, Wesseling H: A double-blind controlled trial of low-dose acetylsalicylic acid and dipyridamole in the treatment of Raynaud's phenomenon. *VASA* (Suppl) 18:71, 1987.

Van der Meulen J, Wouda AA, Mandema E, The TH: Immune complexes in peripheral blood polymorphonuclear leucocytes of patients with Raynaud's phenomenon. *Clin Exp Immunol* 35:62, 1979.

Van de Wal HJCM, Wijn PFF, van Lier HJJ, Skotnicki SH: Quantitative study of the effects of ketanserin in patients with primary Raynaud's phenomenon. *Microcirc Endothel Lymph* 2:657, 1985.

Van Heereveld H, Wollersheim H, Gough K, Thien T: Intravenous nicardipine in Raynaud's phenomenon: a controlled trial. *J Cardiovasc Pharmacol* 11:68, 1988.

Van Wijk TW: The treatment of peripheral vascular diseases with Cyclospasmol. *Angiology* 4:103, 1953.

Varadi DP, Lawrence AM: Suppression of Raynaud's phenomenon by methyldopa. *Ann Intern Med* 124:13, 1969.

Vasko JS, Evans WE: Hemodynamic effects of intravenous alcohol on patients with ischemic limb disease. *J Surg Res* 20:477, 1976.

Vayssairat M, Capron L, Fiessinger J, Mathieu J, Housset E: Calcium channel blockers and Raynaud's disease. *Ann Intern Med* 95:243, 1981.

Waldo R: Prazosin relieves Raynaud's vasospasm. *JAMA* 241:1137, 1979.

Wasner C, Cooke R, Fries JF: Successful medical treatment of scleroderma renal crisis. *N Engl J Med* 299:873, 1978.

Wesseling H, den Heeten A, Wouda AA: Sublingual and oral isoxsuprine in patients with Raynaud's phenomenon. *Eur J Clin Pharmacol* 20:329, 1981.

Wigley FM, Wise RA, Malamet R, Scott TE: Nicardipine in the treatment of Raynaud's phenomenon. *Arthritis Rheum* 30:281, 1987.

Wilgis EFS: Evaluation and treatment of chronic digital ischemia. *Ann Surg* 193:693, 1981.

Willerson JT, Thompson RH, Hookman P, Herdt J, Decker JL: Reserpine in Raynaud's disease and phenomenon. *Ann Intern Med* 72:17, 1970.

Williams HG, Furst DE, Dahl SL, Steen VD, Mark C, Alpert EJ, Henderson AM, Samuelson CO Jr, Drefus JN, Weinstein A, MacLaughlin EJ, Alarcon GS, Kaplan SB, Guttadauria M, Luggen ME, Reading JC, Egger MJ, Ward JR: Double-blind, multicenter controlled trial comparing topical dimethyl sulfoxide and normal saline for treatment of hand ulcers in patients with systemic sclerosis. *Arthritis Rheum* 28:308, 1985.

Winston EL, Pariser KM, Miller KB, Salem DN, Creager MA: Nifedipine as a therapeutic modality for Raynaud's phenomenon. *Arthritis Rheum* 26:1177, 1983.

Wise RA, Malamet R, Wigley FM: Acute effects of nifedipine on digital blood flow in human subjects with Raynaud's phenomenon: a double blind placebo controlled trial. *J Rheumatol* 14:278, 1987.

Wollersheim H, Thien T, Fennis J, van Elteren P, van't Laar A: Double-blind, placebo-controlled study of prazosin in Raynaud's phenomenon. *Clin Pharmacol Ther* 40:219, 1986.

Wollersheim H, Thien T, van't Laar A: Nifedipine in primary Raynaud's phenomenon and in scleroderma: oral versus sublingual hemodynamic effects. *J Clin Pharmacol* 27:907, 1987.

Wong WH, Freedman RI, Rabens SF, Schwartz S, Levan NE: Low molecular weight dextran therapy for scleroderma. *Arch Dermatol* 110:419, 1974.

Yocum DE, Hodes R, Sundstrom WR, Cleeland CS: Use of biofeedback training in treatment of Raynaud's disease and phenomenon. *J Rheumatol* 12:90, 1985.

Zahavi J, Hamilton WAP, O'Reilly MJG, Leyton J, Cotton LT, Kakkar VV: Plasma exchange and platelet function in Raynaud's phenomenon. *Thromb Res* 19:85, 1980.

Zook EG, Kleinert HE, Van Beek AL: Treatment of the ischemic finger secondary to digital artery occlusions. Plast Reconstr Surg 62:229, 1978.

8

Acrocyanosis and Livedo Reticularis

Acrocyanosis and livedo reticularis may share some characteristics with Raynaud's phenomenon. Livedo reticularis is commonly present in patients with primary Raynaud's disease. The benign forms of acrocyanosis and livedo reticularis are reversible by warming the affected parts, suggesting either increased sympathetic nervous system activity or local sensitivity of blood vessels to cold. However, they are distinct clinical entities that must be differentiated from Raynaud's phenomenon. Patients with idiopathic acrocyanosis have persistently blue digits, hands, and feet, and all digits are affected. Livedo reticularis most commonly occurs on the extremities but may involve the trunk of the body. Patients with Raynaud's phenomenon have episodic attacks of well demarcated color changes confined to the digits. If cyanosis occurs, only the digits are involved, and the coloring is well demarcated, not diffuse. The episodic attacks do not always involve all fingers, and often the thumbs are spared. With Raynaud's phenomenon vasospasm occurs at the level of the digital arteries (see Chap. 4), whereas with acrocyanosis and livedo reticularis it is probable that the vasoconstriction occurs in small blood vessels such as the arterioles. Acrocyanosis can also occur whenever blood flow is slow, allowing the hemoglobin to lose much of its oxygen. Therefore all three entities may be present in patients with connective tissue diseases. It is not uncommon for patients with scleroderma to have persistently cyanotic fingers and hands as well as to experience attacks of blanching of the fingers.

ACROCYANOSIS

Crocq in 1896 described patients whose hands and feet slowly became blue, with the discoloration ending gradually at the wrist and dorsum of the foot on exposures to cool or cold environments. The discoloration was deeper on the volar surfaces, and local pressure caused a white area that slowly disappeared. Edema, ulceration, paresis, severe pain, or contractures did not occur. Idiopathic acrocyanosis can be defined as persistent coldness and cyanosis of the digits, hands, and feet sometimes extending proximally to the arms; it is intensified by exposure to cold (Peacock, 1957; Stern, 1937). Stern (1937) found that edema occurred in the more severe cases, sweating of the palms and soles was common, and the face and ears were sometimes involved. Acrocyanosis is usually considered a benign disorder and should not be confused with the persistent, diffuse cyanosis of the digits, hands, and feet that occurs on cold exposure in some patients with scleroderma and other connective tissue diseases. It is questionable if the patients studied by Peacock (1957, 1959) had idiopathic acrocyanosis, as symptoms were severe enough in eight patients to require sympathectomy.

Secondary acrocyanosis may occur in association with the connective tissue diseases or any disease with central cyanosis. A 5-year-old boy with infectious mononucleosis and persistent acrocyanosis of the tongue, nose, lips, fingers, and toes due to cold agglutinins has been described (Dickerman et al., 1980). His serum contained anti-M and anti-I antibodies, and his red blood cells agglutinated in the cold. Edwards (1956) described 20 patients with symmetrical cyanosis, coldness, and pain in the hands and feet. The onset appeared suddenly and lasted several months without a seasonal variation. Necrosis of the tips of the fingers and toes often occurred in these patients, who were in their sixth to eighth decades. Biopsies of the skin showed partial or complete obstruction by intimal proliferation of arterioles and small arteries. Perivascular inflammation with lymphocytes was present, and hyaline thrombi frequently occluded the capillaries in the dermis. No common precipitating cause was found, both male and female patients were afflicted, and all the extremities were involved in 11 patients.

Pathology

Only one study has been reported on the pathology of idiopathic acrocyanosis. Stern (1937) examined skin sections from the dorsum of the hands and feet of 12 patients and compared them to sections from normal controls. The medial layer of the arterioles was thickened, measuring 30 to 150 μm in diameter. Sometimes the number of nuclei were increased, suggesting proliferation of muscle fibers. These changes may have been within the upper limits seen in the normal specimens. However, there was also local edema and fibrosis of the skin; and considerable dilatation of the superficial capillaries was sometimes found.

Etiology

The etiology of idiopathic acrocyanosis is unknown. Stern (1937) considered that inactivity led to cold sensitivity; the patients he studied were all in a mental hospital. Crocq (1896) mentioned that two of his patients had hysteria.

Pathophysiology

Lewis and Landis (1930) surmised that there was no venous obstruction, as elevation of the cyanotic limb above the heart produced pallor, and the pallor induced by pressure disappeared spontaneously. A red area appeared in the cyanosis after trauma. With body heating, the temperature of the fingers reached that of the forehead, and reactive hyperemia of the fingers was normal, ruling against structural disease of the vessels. Ulnar nerve block relieved the cyanosis of the fifth finger. The color did not change until the temperature of the digit rose 7°C, which was interpreted to mean that the digital arteries opened before "spasm" was relieved in the arterioles. Vasoconstrictor agents produced a normal response in acrocyanotic hands. This indirect evidence for arteriolar vasospasm was confirmed by the studies of Eliot and co-workers (1936) and Lambie and Morson (1937). Larsson (1948) described a poorly defined group of patients with "acroasphyxia" who had a high peripheral vascular tone determined by a lower skin temperature than normal subjects and a prolonged time to vasodilatation during body and local heating. Peacock (1957, 1959) reported that his patients had hand blood flows (plethysmography) in the normal range during local warming to 42°C but had low blood flow and skin temperature at 32°C. The latter flows were in the same range found in patients with primary Raynaud's disease. One of the most interesting studies described a 6.5-year-old girl whose intensely cyanotic hands and forearms became warm and red during sleep (Day and Klingman, 1939). There was a prompt rise in finger and hand skin temperature with normal sleep; and cooling and cyanosis occurred upon awakening. During phenobarbital-induced sleep, the hands responded in the same manner as the rest of the body to heat and cold exposures. The investigators considered these findings strong evidence for an abnormal vasomotor response of central origin and against a local sensitivity of the blood vessels to cold.

There are many descriptions in the literature indicating that the nailfold capillary loops, especially on the venous side, are dilated; and the spontaneous velocity of the red blood cells has been found to be decreased (Day and Klingman, 1939; Meier et al., 1978). Jacobs and co-workers (1987) found that the number of capillaries was decreased, and there were larger capillary loops in their patients compared to those in normal subjects and patients with primary Raynaud's disease. They also reported a decrease in red blood cell velocity after cold provocation. The capillary flow is not homogeneous in that some capillaries show intermittent flow adjacent to capillaries with continuous flow (Bollinger et al., 1977). Delayed and asynchronous arrival of fluorescein sodium in different capillaries corroborated this finding (Franzeck et al., 1983). With a cold stimulus, inhomogeneous capillary flow patterns persisted contrary to findings in normal subjects.

Incidence, Sex, Age

The incidence of acrocyanosis is unknown. There is no sex predominance. The age range has been reported as 20 to 45 years (Stern, 1937).

Clinical Picture

Patients usually present with bluish digits, hands, feet, and sometimes forearms that sweat excessively. The discoloration intensifies on cold exposure consistently and during emotional upsets occasionally; heating causes the return of normal color or redness to the involved areas. Except for mild digital swelling, trophic changes and pain do not occur. Physical examination is normal, and all pulses are present. No changes occur in the hemogram or erythrocyte sedimentation rate (ESR); antinuclear antibodies are not present.

Differential Diagnosis

The main differential diagnosis is Raynaud's phenomenon. However, the hands and feet are not involved in patients with Raynaud's phenomenon. With acrocyanosis, the color change is persistent, not episodic; the cyanosis of the digits is not well demarcated; and a pallor phase does not occur. Primary Raynaud's disease affects predominantly female subjects, whereas acrocyanosis has no sex predilection. With acrocyanosis the nailbed capillaries are moderately enlarged, discordant flow patterns are more frequent, and there is less decrease in red blood cell velocity than in primary Raynaud's disease (Bollinger, 1985). Acrocyanosis due to connective tissue diseases can be differentiated by history, physical examination, and appropriate laboratory tests (see Chap. 6). Central cyanosis can be diagnosed by an arterial oxygen saturation determination.

Treatment

Treatment is usually unnecessary for this benign disease. Patients often complain of the cosmetic problem of bluish, moist hands that can be a social embarrassment. For the few patients who request therapy, small doses of adrenergic blocking agents (reserpine, guanethidine) have been successful in our experience.

Summary

Acrocyanosis is an entity whose pathology, pathophysiology, or clinical spectrum has not been adequately defined. In the idiopathic form, it is a benign disease without severe symptoms or trophic changes. The hands, feet, and digits are persistently blue, cold, and moist; normal color returns with warming of the part. Swelling of the digits may occur. Physical examination, except for the cyanosis and coldness, is normal, as are laboratory tests. There are indications of decreased blood flow in the hands and digital capillaries, with nonhomogeneous flow on cold exposure compared to that in normal subjects. Both sexes are affected during the third to fifth decades. The differential diagnosis from Raynaud's phenomenon should not be difficult as the color change is not episodic, well demarcated, or confined to the digits. Treatment is usually unnecessary. Acrocyanosis may occur secondary to connective tissue diseases or any disease that markedly decreases blood flow. It is also seen in conjunction with any disease that causes central cyanosis.

LIVEDO RETICULARIS

Livedo reticularis has been called by many names, including asphyxia reticularis, livedo racemosa, livedo annularis, cutis marmorata, idiopathic livedo reticularis, and sympathetic livedo reticularis. The most commonly used appellations for livedo reticularis with ulceration are livedo vasculitis, livedoid vasculitis, and atrophie blanche. The variety of names reflects the unknown etiology of the disease.

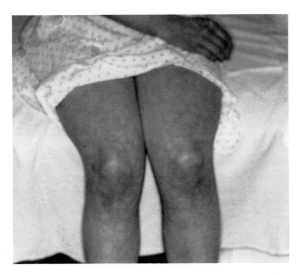

Fig. 8–1. Lacelike, or fishnet, pattern of livedo reticularis on the lower extremities of a young woman. This patient had no symptoms or signs of a secondary disease. The webs of the fishnet can be rose, violet red, or blue; the skin between the webs is normal or pale.

Livedo reticularis with ulceration was originally described by Milian (1929) as *atrophie blanche en plaque;* he considered it a manifestation of syphilis.

Classification

1. Livedo reticularis in its benign form is a mottled discoloration of the extremities and sometimes the trunk of the body in a reticular, fishnet, or lacelike pattern (Fig. 8–1). It is reversible by exposure to a warm environment and aggravated by cold.
2. Livedo reticularis with ulceration is a form of vasculitis or vascular thrombosis. The skin pattern is the same as in the benign form but is usually irreversible.
3. Secondary livedo reticularis may be seen in association with several diseases, especially the connective tissue diseases, and with drug treatment. The mechanism of this secondary disease may be related to that of the benign form or the vasculitic form.

Pathology

With the benign, reversible form of livedo reticularis and that due to drug therapy, biopsy results are either nonspecific (Pearce et al., 1974) or show an increased number of dilated capillaries (Barker et al., 1941). In livedo reticularis with ulceration, a segmental hyalinizing vasculitis is seen that mainly affects the middle dermal vessels. The vessel walls are thickened with or without lymphocytic cuffing; hyaline degeneration and areas of focal thrombosis are present. Hemorrhages and new vessel proliferation may occur. Papillary and deeper dermal vessels may also be involved (Barker et al., 1941; Cabbabe and Clift, 1985; Feldaker, 1956; Schroeter et al., 1975). In patients with ulcerations, infarcts of the skin are caused by obstructed arterioles.

Pathophysiology

The fishnet appearance of the skin in livedo reticularis is compatible with vasospasm or obstruction of the small perpendicular arterioles that lie in the dermis. The red to blue periphery of each web of the net can be explained by deoxygenated blood in the surrounding horizontally arranged venous plexuses (Williams and Goodman, 1925). Copeland (1975) argued strongly for the color changes being due to stasis of blood in the superficial veins of the skin. Support for this mechanism derives from the fact that elevation of the extremity decreases the intensity of the color changes probably by draining the veins. With the benign form of livedo reticularis, the reversibility of the color pattern with warming, the frequent association with vasospastic diseases of the digits, and the response to sympathetic blocking agents suggests increased sympathetic nervous system activity as the cause.

The nature of the pathological findings has led investigators to ascribe livedo reticularis with ulceration to a localized vasculitis (Winkelmann et al., 1974). Immunofluorescence studies have demonstrated mainly immunoglobulin M (IgM) deposits; complement factors, fibrin, and sometimes IgA have also been found in the vessel walls, suggesting an immune complex pathogenesis. These findings are similar to those seen with some of the connective tissue diseases.

Matsuda and co-workers (1976) documented a complex of fibrinogen and a cold insoluble globulin in the plasma of four patients with skin ulcers of the legs. Three of the four patients developed their ulcerations during the winter. Livedo reticularis was not described in these patients, but a cryoprotein may be of etiological importance in some patients with recurrent leg ulcerations.

Other investigators consider this disease may be due to blood or tissue abnormalities leading to thromboses of arterioles instead of a vasculitis. Decreased fibrinolytic activity has been found in the tissues of lesions of ulcerated limbs (Cunliffe and Menon, 1971), and the average plasma level of releasable vascular (tissue-type) plasminogen activator was reported to be markedly decreased compared to that in control subjects (Pizzo et al., 1986). Therefore there may be a defect in the fibrinolytic system. This possibility has led to the use of agents that enhance fibrinolytic activity in treatment. Although these agents cause clinical improvement in some patients, they often fail. Other investigators report abnormalities of platelet aggregation e.g., hyperaggregation of platelets with epinephrine, adenosine diphosphate, or collagen or increased platelet adhesiveness (Drucker and Duncan, 1982; Yamamoto et al., 1988). Correction of these abnormalities with antiplatelet agents has led to alleviation of the syndrome but only in some patients. Such defects in the fibrinolytic system or in platelets could cause the thrombotic occlusion of dermal vessels, but whether these abnormalities are primary or secondary is unknown.

Milstone and colleagues (1983) postulated that atrophie blanche with or without livedo reticularis is due to occlusion rather than inflammation of vessels in the middle and deep dermis. Their patients were predominantly female but were more elderly than in other reports. However, inflammatory cells were often present in their biopsy specimens in addition to dilated or occluded vessels, so an initial vasculitis could not be ruled out. They considered that reduced blood flow in the subpapillary venous plexus in the areas of livedo reticularis could induce vascular occlusion and hence atrophie blanche, or that alterations in local blood flow from occlusion of vessels could cause livedo reticularis.

Amantadine causes livedo reticularis and is known to release norepinephrine from central and peripheral nerve terminals in addition to enhancing the action of norepinephrine and dopamine on several peripheral tissues (Heimans et al., 1972). It may also inhibit uptake of dopamine and norepinephrine in neurons. All of these actions could lead to arteriolar vasoconstriction. Pearce and co-workers (1974) have shown decreased limb blood flow in three of five patients and decreased skin temperature in four of five patients during amantadine treatment.

Incidence, Sex, Age

The incidence of these conditions is unknown, but livedo reticularis is common in young women. Livedo reticularis with ulceration is rare. Benign livedo reticularis occurs mostly in women during the second to fifth decades of life. Livedo reticularis with ulceration is most common in women (Winkelmann et al., 1974) but is seen not infrequently in men (Barker et al., 1941). The onset has been reported in patients from 9 to 80 years of age, but most cases present in the 20- to 45-year age group.

Clinical Picture

With the benign form, the webs of the fishnet are a rose, violet, red, or blue color. Between the webs the skin appears normal but pale. The extremities are mainly afflicted, and there may be subjective or objective coldness of the skin. Except for numbness and rarely pain (Barker et al., 1941), other symptoms do not occur. The color pattern is aggravated by cold exposure and may disappear on warming. In our experience, it is a common condition in the general population, almost always asymptomatic, and often associated with primary Raynaud's disease or acrocyanosis.

In those with livedo reticularis and ulceration, the fishnet pattern of the skin is usually persistent and not relieved by warming, but it is exacerbated by cold. Purpuric macular lesions and cutaneous nodules develop and progress to ulcers often covered with eschars and bordered by an inflammatory response. These ulcers may occur only during the winter months, although some patients are more apt to develop them during the summer (Feldaker et al., 1956). They are painful and usually take months to heal. Edema occurs in 50 percent of patients often 1 to 2 weeks before ulceration appears. Healed ulcers leave a smooth ivory-white plaque of atrophic skin surrounded by hyperpigmented borders and telangiectatic blood vessels (atrophie blanche) (Fig. 8–2). Most ulcers occur on the lower part of the legs, ankles, and dorsum of the feet. In patients with ulcers only during the winter,

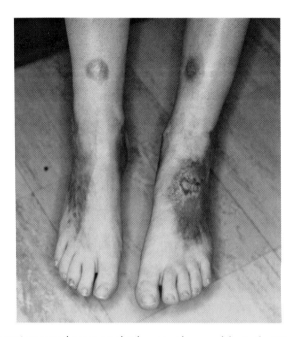

Fig. 8–2. Hyperpigmented scars on the lower calves and feet of a 27-year-old woman who has had recurrent ulcerations for 15 years. This entity is often referred to as "atrophie blanche." The patient has had multiple work-ups for secondary disease with no abnormal physical findings, except on the lower extremities, and no abnormal laboratory tests. Even with active ulcers and inflammation, her white blood cell count and ESR were normal.

hypertension, Raynaud's phenomenon, acrocyanosis, and digital arterial thromboses were found to be more common, whereas edema of the legs and feet was a more prominent feature in patients with summer ulcerations (Feldaker et al., 1956).

Secondary livedo reticularis may be benign or ulcerative. Amandatine hydrochloride causes the benign form, which occurs frequently in patients being treated for Parkinson's disease (Pearce et al., 1974; Shealy et al., 1970). It affects both sexes, is more prominent on the legs, and is often accompanied by pedal edema. It usually disappears within 2 to 6 weeks if the drug is discontinued, although its presence is not a reason for stopping the medication (Silver and Sahs, 1972). Livedo reticularis has been reported in association with connective tissue diseases, polyarteritis nodosa, vasculitis, obstructive arterial diseases, endocrine disorders, infections, neurogenic diseases, hyperviscosity states, cryoglobulinemias, thrombocythemia, lymphomas, and atheromatous microembolism (Copeman, 1975). Sneddon (1965) described a syndrome of livedo reticularis with cerebrovascular lesions; two other groups of investigators have documented the seriousness of this disease (Rebollo et al., 1983; Rumpl et al., 1985). Patients have extensive livedo reticularis over the body and transient ischemic attacks or strokes. Cerebral angiograms have shown thromboses or no disease. Hughes (1984) described a subgroup of patients with lupus erythematosus who had arterial or venous thromboses, spontaneous abortions, anticardiolipin antibodies, and livedo reticularis. Weinstein and co-workers (1987) found that 38 of 78 patients with lupus erythematosus had livedo reticularis. There was a significant association of moderate to severe livedo reticularis with elevated levels of anticardiolipin antibodies. Two of their patients with cerebral infarcts and severe livedo reticularis could be classified as Sneddon's syndrome. These patients did not develop other features of lupus erythematosus until 3 and 10 years later. Weinstein and co-workers proposed that anticardiolipin antibodies may be the cause of Sneddon's syndrome and precede other clinical and laboratory manifestations of lupus erythematosus. Livedo reticularis evidently can occur whenever there is decreased blood flow to the skin due to either vascular obstruction, sludging of blood, or neurogenic vasoconstriction. The appearance of livedo reticularis may be a clue to the diagnosis of some diseases, e.g., microembolism and hyperviscosity syndromes.

The physical examination of patients without secondary disease is normal except for the extremity lesions. Arterial pulses are normal.

Laboratory Tests

Except in the patients with livedo reticularis due to secondary diseases, there are no consistently abnormal laboratory tests for livedo reticularis or livedo reticularis with ulceration (Winkelmann et al., 1974). In our experience, even the ESR and white blood cell count have been normal in the presence of multiple ulcerations on the lower limbs. Antinuclear antibodies and rheumatoid factor testing help in the diagnosis of the connective tissue diseases.

Prognosis

The prognosis of the benign condition is excellent; it is often only a cosmetic problem, especially in fair-skinned women. Livedo reticularis with ulceration has a poor prognosis because of recurrent, painful ulcerations of the lower extremities, but it does not cause other morbidity or mortality. Ulcers are often recurrent for up to 20 years (Cabbabe and Clift, 1985; Coffman, personal observations). The lower limbs and feet may become scarred, and amputations have been necessary for deep ulcers and severe pain (Barker et al., 1941; Cabbabe and Clift, 1985).

Treatment

The benign type of livedo reticularis needs no treatment. In young women bothered by the social stigma of the skin discoloration, we have had good success with small doses of reserpine (0.125–0.250 mg daily). Treatment for livedo reticularis due to other diseases is that of the underlying disease and is often successful.

Unfortunately, livedo reticularis with ulceration has not been responsive to the usual treatments for immune complex diseases. The mainstay of treatment has been saline soaks and analgesic ointment. If edema is present, limbs should be elevated above heart level, as tissue swelling interferes with healing.

Because a defect in the fibrinolytic system and abnormalities in platelet aggregation have been demonstrated in patients with livedo reticularis with ulcerations, fibrinolysis-promoting and antiplatelet agents have been used. Phenformin with ethylestrenol or stanozolol have been given to induce fibrinolysis with reportedly good results (Basler and Jones, 1978; Gilliam et al., 1974; Milstone et al., 1983). Ethylestrenol does not benefit patients when used alone, and phenformin is no longer available because it may induce lactic acidosis. Aspirin, dipyridamole, and triclopidine, alone or in combination, have also improved some patients (Drucker and Duncan, 1982; Yamamoto et al., 1988). However, each of these therapies has proved unsuccessful in some patients, and recurrences are common. Intravenous infusions of low-molecular-weight dextran for 4 weeks have been reported to promote healing and decrease the number of relapses (Issroff and Whiting, 1971). Dextran increases skin blood flow probably by plasma volume expansion, coating of platelets, and reducing red blood cell sludging.

Nicotinic acid, 300 to 500 mg daily, was reported in one study to benefit 9 of 12 patients and to make one patient worse (Winkelmann et al., 1974). Six patients with atrophie blanche were improved, although not cured by pentoxyfylline (Sauer, 1986), and one patient responded to nifedipine after failing with aspirin and dipyridamole (Purcell and Hayes, 1986). One patient also improved with minidose heparin (Jetton and Lazarus, 1983). Corticosteroids, cytoxan, methotrexate, salicylates, sulfa drugs, antibiotics, griseofulvin, β-adrenoceptor antagonists, and radiotherapy have been tried with little success. Occasional patients have responded to each therapy. Sympathetic blocking agents have also been used. Hexamethonium or guanethidine has helped some patients (Winkelmann et al., 1974). Tindall and co-workers (1974) gave four to eight intraarterial injections of 1.0 to 3.0 mg of reserpine and obtained complete clearing of lesions in two of three patients. Surgical sympathectomy has not proved to be of long-term benefit (Barker et al., 1941).

If a disease is being treated with multiple forms of therapy, it is clear that its cause is unknown and there is as yet no successful treatment. Such is the case here. Fibrinolysis-promoting and antiplatelet agents currently appear to be most popular, but they do not lead to complete or lasting remissions. Without controlled studies, it is difficult to evaluate these forms of therapy, as patients often have spontaneous remissions. Moreover, we have cared for patients who did not respond to any of the proposed therapies. One of our patients had a complete remission for her entire pregnancy; and it was her first prolonged period without ulcers. An extensive endocrinological work-up was completely normal.

Summary

Livedo reticularis is a lacelike discoloration of the extremities and sometimes the trunk of the body. It may occur in a benign form on exposure to cold, may accompany vasospastic conditions, and is usually asymptomatic. Amandatine can cause a similar condition. Livedo reticularis with painful ulcerations (or atrophie blanche) is usually a severe, recurrent disease of the lower limbs that occurs during winter or summer and mostly in women. Healing of the ulcers often leaves a white scar with a hyperpigmented border. Laboratory studies are usually normal. Pathological findings suggest either a thrombotic disease or vasculitis. Secondary livedo reticularis may occur in association with many diseases that occlude or slow blood flow through small blood vessels. The benign form of the disease needs no treatment. Therapy for livedo reticularis with ulcerations has not been successful, although some patients improve with fibrinolysis-enhancing or antiplatelet agents. Much remains to be learned about livedo reticularis with ulcerations.

REFERENCES

Acrocyanosis

Bollinger A: Function of the precapillary vessels in peripheral vascular disease. *J Cardiovasc Pharmacol* 7(suppl 3):S147, 1985.

Bollinger A, Mahler F, Meier B: Velocity patterns in nailfold capillaries of normal subjects and patients with Raynaud's disease and acrocyanosis. *Bibl Anat* 16:142, 1977.

Crocq C: De l'acrocyanose. *Sem Med* 16:297, 1896.

Day R, Klingman WO: The effect of sleep on the skin temperature reactions in a case of acrocyanosis. *J Clin Invest* 18:271, 1939.

Dickerman JD, Howard P, Dopp S, Staley R: Infectious mononucleosis initially seen as cold-induced acrocyanosis. *Am J Dis Child* 134:159, 1980.

Edwards EE: Remittent necrotizing acrocyanosis. *JAMA* 161:1530, 1956.

Eliot AH, Evans RD, Stone CS: Acrocyanosis: a study of the circulatory fault. *Am Heart J* 11:431, 1936.

Franzeck UK, Isenring G, Frey J, Bollinger A: Videodensitometric pattern recognition of Na-fluorescein diffusion in nailfold capillary areas of patients with acrocyanosis, primary vasospastic and secondary Raynaud's phenomenon. *Int Angiol* 2:143, 1983.

Jacobs MJHM, Breslau PJ, Sloaf DW, Reneman RS, Lemmens JAJ: Nomenclature of Raynaud's phenomenon: a capillary microscopic and hemorheologic study. *Surgery* 101:136, 1987.

Lambie CG, Morson SM: Acrocyanosis. *Med J Aust* 2:1070, 1937.

Larsson Y: The vasoconstrictor tone of the cutaneous arterioles in acroasphyxia, hypertension and in the cold pressor test. *Acta Med Scand* [Suppl 206] 130:146, 1948.

Lewis T, Landis EM: Observations upon the vascular mechanism in acrocyanosis. *Heart* 15:229, 1930.

Meier B, Mahler F, Bollinger A: Blutflussgeschwindigkeit in nagelfalzkapillaren bei gesunden und patienten mit vasospastischen und organischen akralen durchblutungastorungen. *Vasa* 7:194, 1978.

Peacock JH: Vasodilatation in the human hand: observations on primary Raynaud's disease and acrocyanosis of the upper extremities. *Clin Sci* 17:575, 1957.

Peacock JH: A comparative study of the digital cutaneous temperatures, and hand blood flows in the normal hand, primary Raynaud's disease and primary acrocyanosis. *Clin Sci* 18:25, 1959.

Stern ES: The aetiology and pathology of acrocyanosis. *Br J Derm Syph* 49:100, 1937.

Livedo Reticularis

Barker NW, Hines EA Jr, Craig WMcK: Livedo reticularis: a peripheral arteriolar disease. *Am Heart J* 21:592, 1941.

Basler RSW, Jones HE: Phenformin in the treatment of livedo reticularis. *N Engl J Med* 298:281, 1978.

Cabbabe EB, Clift SD: Leg ulcerations in livedoid vasculitis. *Plast Reconstr Surg* 75:888, 1985.

Copeman PWM: Livedo reticularis. *Br J Dermatol* 93:519, 1975.

Cunliffe WJ, Menon IS: The association between cutaneous vasculitis and decreased blood fibrinolytic activity. *Br J Dermatol* 84:99, 1971.

Drucker CR, Duncan WC: Antiplatelet therapy in atrophie blanche and livedo vasculitis. *J Am Acad Dermatol* 7:359, 1982.

Feldaker M, Hines EA Jr, Kierland RR: Livedo reticularis with ulcerations. *Circulation* 13:196, 1956.

Gilliam J, Herndon JH, Prystowsky SD: Fibrinolytic therapy for vasculitis of atrophie blanche. *Arch dermatol* 109:664, 1974.

Heimans RLH, Rand MJ, Fennessy MR: Some actions of amantadine on peripheral tissues. *J Pharm Pharmacol* 24:869, 1972.

Hughes GRV: Autoantibodies in lupus and its variants: experience in 1000 patients. *Br Med J* 289:339, 1984.

Issroff SW, Whiting DA: Low molecular weight dextran in the treatment of livedo reticularis with ulceration. *Br J Dermatol* 85(suppl 7):26, 1971.

Jetton RL, Lazarus GS: Minidose heparin therapy for vasculitis of atrophie blanche. *J Am Acad Dermatol* 8:23, 1983.

Matsuda M, Saida T, Hasegawa R: Cryofibrinogen in the plasma of patients with skin ulcerative lesions on the legs: a complex of fibrinogen and cold insoluble globulin. *Thromb Res* 9:541, 1976.

Milian G: Les atrophies cutanees syphilitiques. *Bull Soc Fr Dermatol Syphigr* 36:865, 1929.

Milstone LM, Braverman IM, Lucky P, Fleckman P: Classification and therapy of atrophie blanche. *Arch Dermatol* 119:963, 1983.

Pearce LA, Waterbury LD, Green HD: Amantadine hydrochloride: alteration in peripheral circulation. *Neurology* 24:46, 1974.

Pizzo SV, Murray JC, Gonias SL: Atrophie blanche: a disorder associated with defective release of tissue plasminogen activator. *Arch Pathol Lab Med* 110:517, 1986.

Purcell SM, Hayes TJ: Nifedipine treatment of idiopathic atrophie blanche. *J Am Acad Dermatol* 14:851, 1986.

Rebollo M, Val JF, Garijo F, Quintana F, Berciano J: Livedo reticularis and cerebrovascular lesions (Sneddon's syndrome). *Brain* 106:965, 1983.

Rumpl E, Neuhofer J, Pallua A, Willeit J, Vogl G, Stampfel G, Platz Th: Cerebrovascular lesions and livedo reticularis (Sneddon's syndrome)—a progressive cerebrovascular disorder? *J Neurol* 231:324, 1985.

Sauer GC: Pentoxifylline (Trental) therapy for the vasculitis of atrophie blanche. *Arch Dermatol* 122:380, 1986.

Schroeter AL, Diaz-Perez JL, Winkelmann RK, Jordan RE: Livedo vasculitis (the vasculitis of atrophie blanche). *Arch Dermatol* 111:188, 1975.

Shealy CN, Weeth JB, Mercier D: Livedo reticularis in patients with parkinsonism receiving amantadine. *JAMA* 212:1522, 1970.

Silver D, Sahs AL: Livedo reticularis in Parkinson's disease patients treated with amantadine hydrochloride. *Neurology* 22:645, 1972.

Sneddon IB: Cerebrovascular lesions and livedo reticularis. *Br J Dermatol* 77:180, 1965.

Tindall JP, Whalen RE, Burton EE Jr: Medical uses of intra-arterial injections of reserpine. *Arch Dermatol* 110:233, 1974.

Weinstein C, Miller MH, Axtens R, Buchanan R, Littlejohn GO: Livedo reticularis associated with increased titers of anticardiolipin antibodies in systemic lupus erythematosus. *Arch Dermatol* 123:596, 1987.

Williams C, Goodman H: Livedo reticularis. *JAMA* 85:955, 1925.

Winkelmann RK, Schroeter AL, Kierland RR, Ryan TM: Clinical studies of livedoid vasculitis (segmental hyalinizing vasculitis). *Mayo Clin Proc* 49:746, 1974.

Yamamoto M, Danno K, Shio H, Imamura S: Antithrombic treatment in livedo vasculitis. *J Am Acad Dermatol* 18:57, 1988.

Index